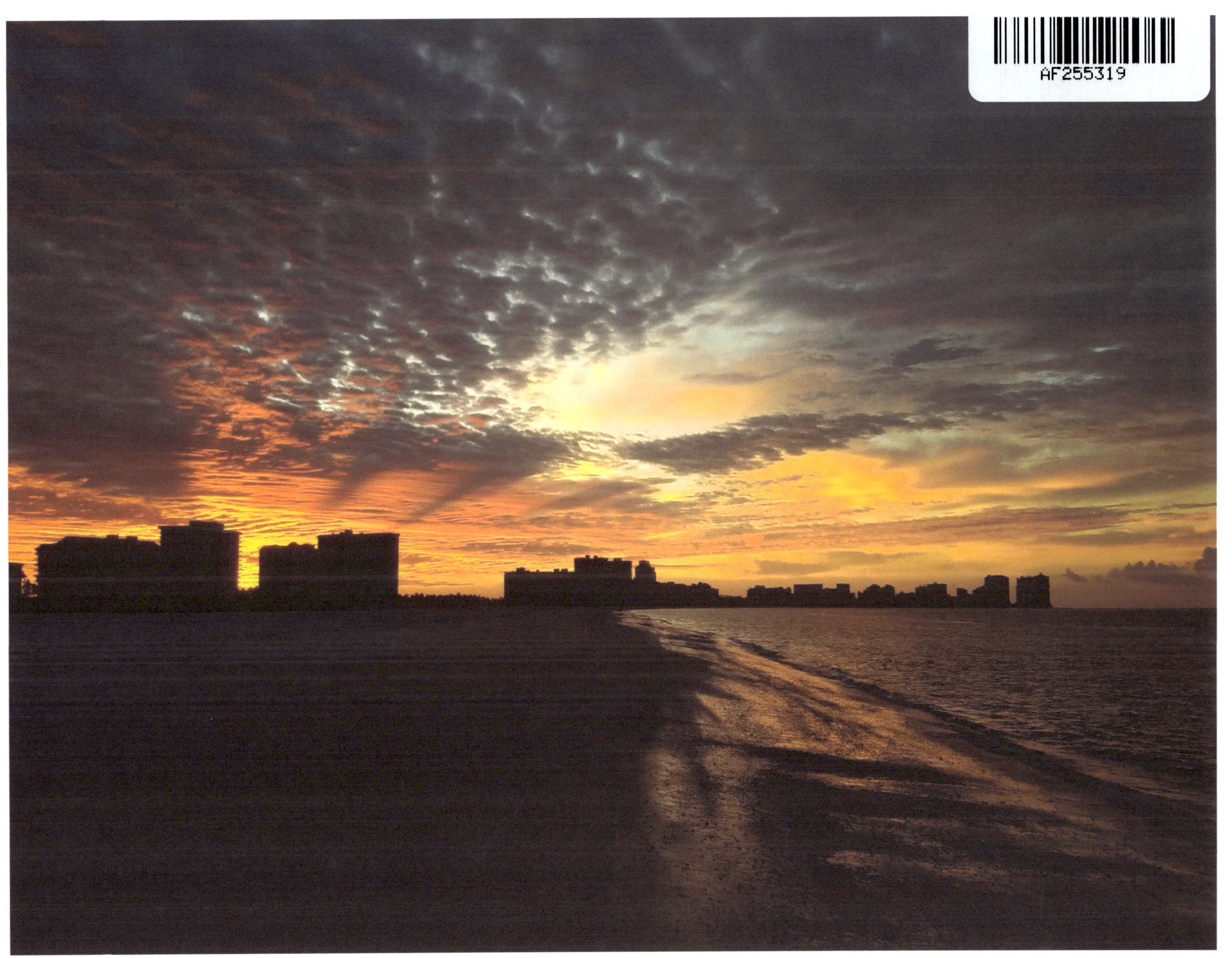
AF255319

Acknowledgements

I'd like to thank Joanne Tailele from Simon Publishing for her help in editing,

designing and formatting this book. Her creative work captured the essence

of what I was trying to portray. It is truly a work of art thanks to her.

Table of Contents

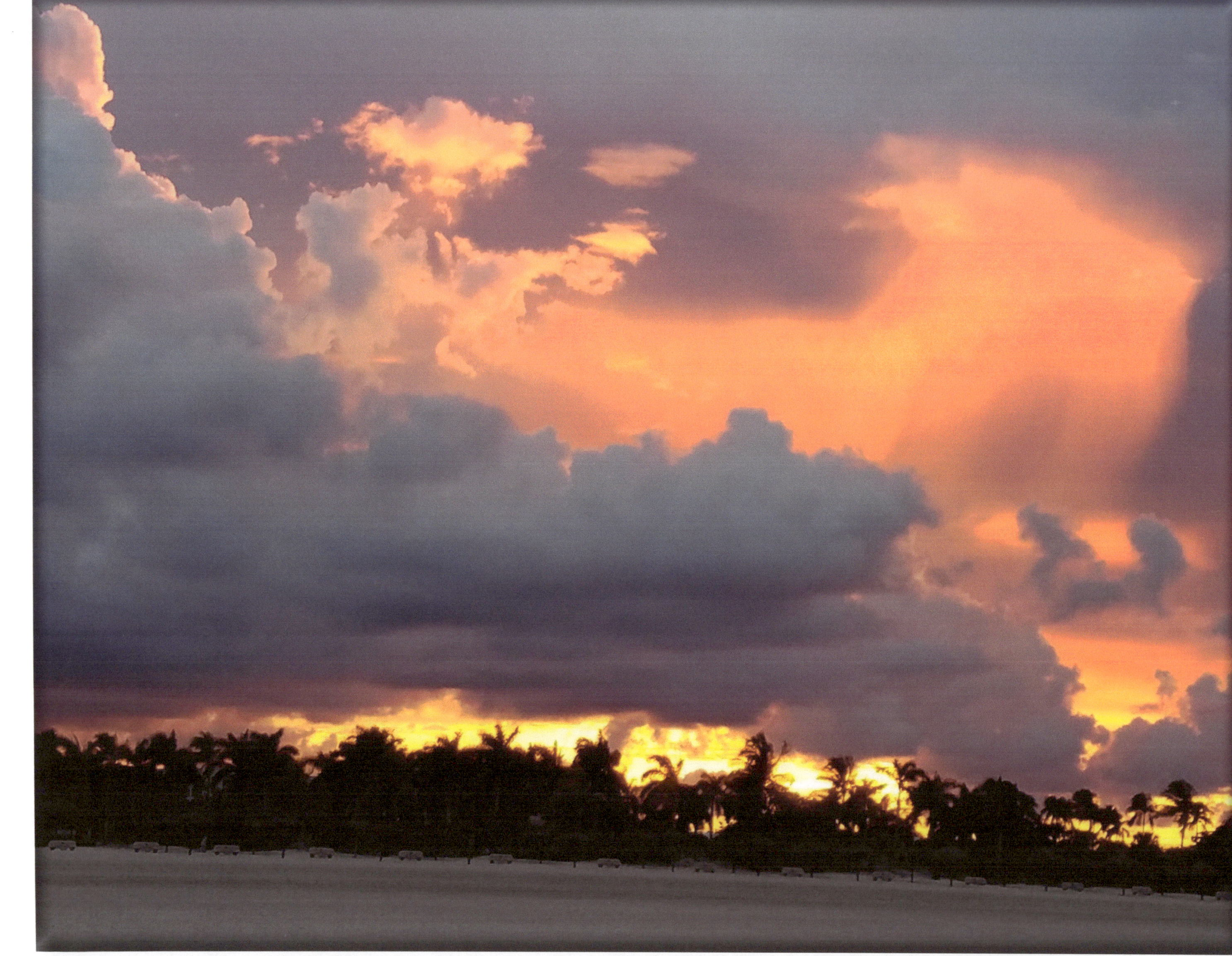

I wrote this book for two reasons; (1) to share with you my passion for watching the sun rise over Marco Island's beautiful waterways and (2) to show you how to enrich your life with mindfulness. I am blessed to live on Marco Island full time and experience its beautiful sunrises almost every day. All of the photos in this book were taken during my sunrise runs on the beach or kayak outings in the 10,000 islands. Marco Island is the first and largest of the 10,000 islands that stretch all the way along the Gulf of Mexico to Key West.

Mindfulness is all about paying attention to the present moment with all five of your senses. Practicing mindfulness will not only increase your awareness of the beauty and uniqueness of Marco Island, it will deepen your connection to all of the things in your life that truly resonate for you. Some of the things about life on Marco Island that really resonate with me are running and meditating on the beach and kayaking. I love to do all three of those things at sunrise.

Mindfulness enhances these connections for me. For example, when I run mindfully on the beach at sunrise, I am fully aware of the way the sand feels against my feet as I run along the water's edge. I also feel the warm wind washing over me as it blows in from the Gulf of Mexico. When I kayak into the rising sun over Addison Bay, I see the ever-changing horizon fill the sky and clouds with all of the colors of the rainbow. When I meditate on the beach, I hear the waves gently crashing on the shore and the birds singing to each other as they cruise the shoreline looking for breakfast. Whether I am running or kayaking I can sometimes taste the salt in the misty air as it mingles with my sweat and rolls down my face and into my lips.

Practicing mindfulness has helped me become more aware of these sensual connections. This is a blessing that I'd love to share with you and help you attain for yourself.

Affirming what resonates for you is an exercise in faith and can't be proven empirically, you just believe it to be true. You don't need to explain it, justify it, or prove it to anyone else; it just exists inside of you and is a source of great comfort and joy. For example, when I am on the water or at the beach at 6:00 a.m. paddling or running as the sun comes up, I have faith that everything in my life is the way it should be. I feel a spiritual connection to the earth, the water, the sky, and the universe. This connection is not something that I can explain rationally, for what civilized human intentionally gets up at 5:00 a.m. to go run on the beach or paddle off into the darkness to watch the sunrise? If you've experienced the same thing don't worry, you don't have to explain it to anyone, just hand them this book and let them vicariously experience it themselves.

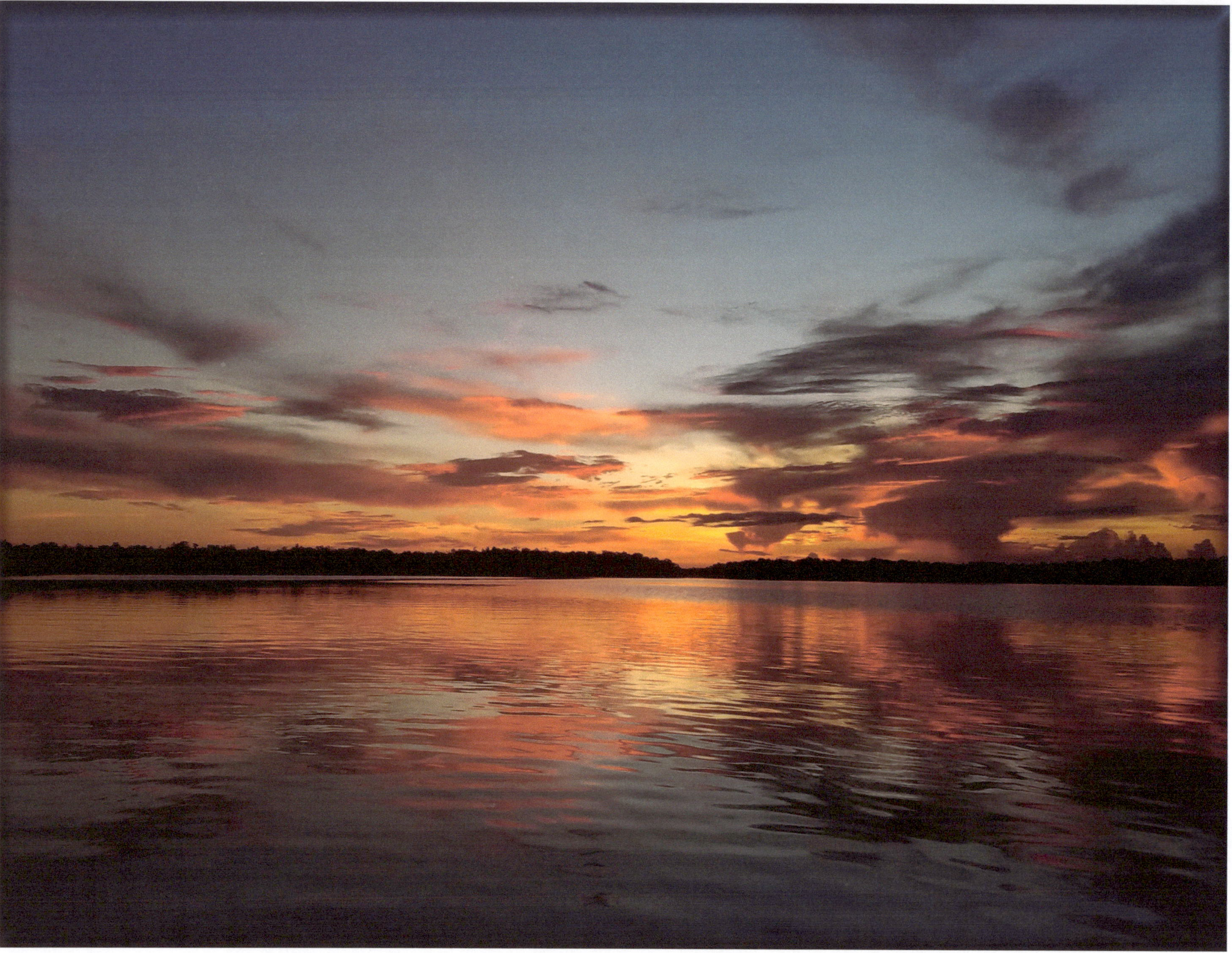

Simply put, Mindfulness is being fully aware of the present moment using all five of your senses. There are four dimensions of mindful moments.

All mindful moments are:

- present centered
- non-conceptual
- non-judgmental
- non-verbal

Mindful moments are present centered because they always focus on the present, never the past or the future. Most of your thoughts are one step removed from the present moment because they focus on the past or future.

Mindful moments are non-conceptual because during them you merely notice what is going on and your thoughts and feelings related to it. You don't try to figure anything out, you simply notice and accept what is going on.

Mindful moments are non-judgmental because they are based on accepting reality for what it is. You do not judge or compare a person or an experience against some arbitrary standard, you just accept them for what they are.

Lastly, mindful moments are non-verbal. They do not involve talking. Speaking involves another layer of cognitive activity that takes you out of the present moment.

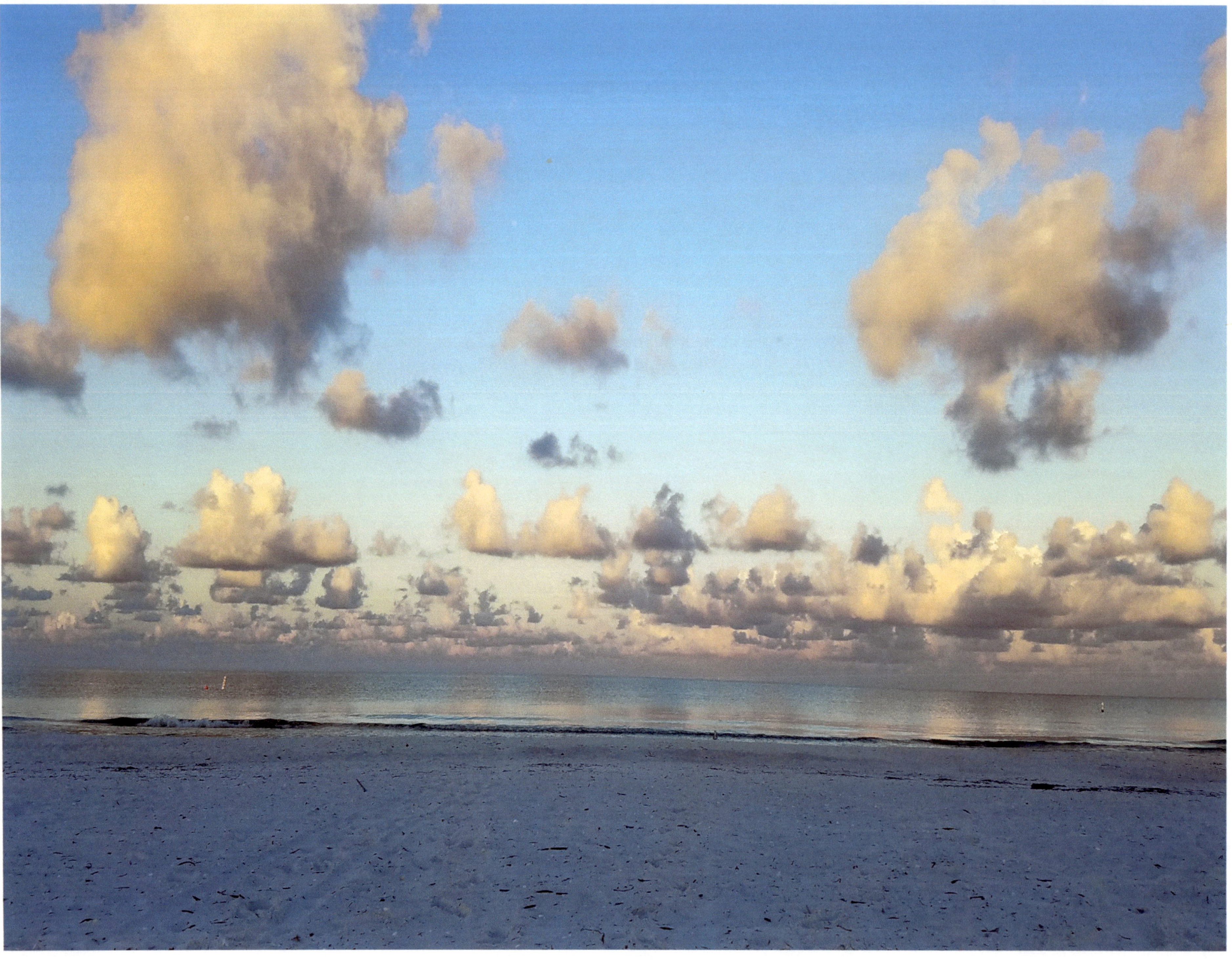

Look at the photo on the opposite page and imagine yourself being there. If you were there and fully involved in the present moment what would it be like? Would you notice the shadows in the clouds as the sun bounced off of the water? Would you feel the sand caress your feet or the breeze gently blow over your body? Would you smell the salt air and taste its residue as it accumulates on your lips? Would you hear the lapping of the waves as they rolled into shore or the gentle cry of the plovers as the skittered up the beach?

Or, would you be thinking about that argument you had with your spouse before you drove off this morning?

Perhaps your mind would be rehashing that meeting you had at work yesterday. It would be going back and forth about what you said, how it was received by your co-workers, what they said, and how you should have responded etc., etc.,

Maybe your mind was jumping ahead to later in the morning after you got off of the water. Would you have time to get home, shower, get dressed and rush off to work? Where would you stop to grab something to eat on the road? What would you eat? Would that conflict with your dinner plans?

While your mind was jumping back and forth from the past to the present and into the future, you missed the sun peek through the clouds and cast a beautiful burst of yellow/orange that only lasted a few seconds.

Unfortunately, because you drifted out of the present moment you lost that image forever for the present moment is fleeting and if you do not pay attention to it, it passes you by.

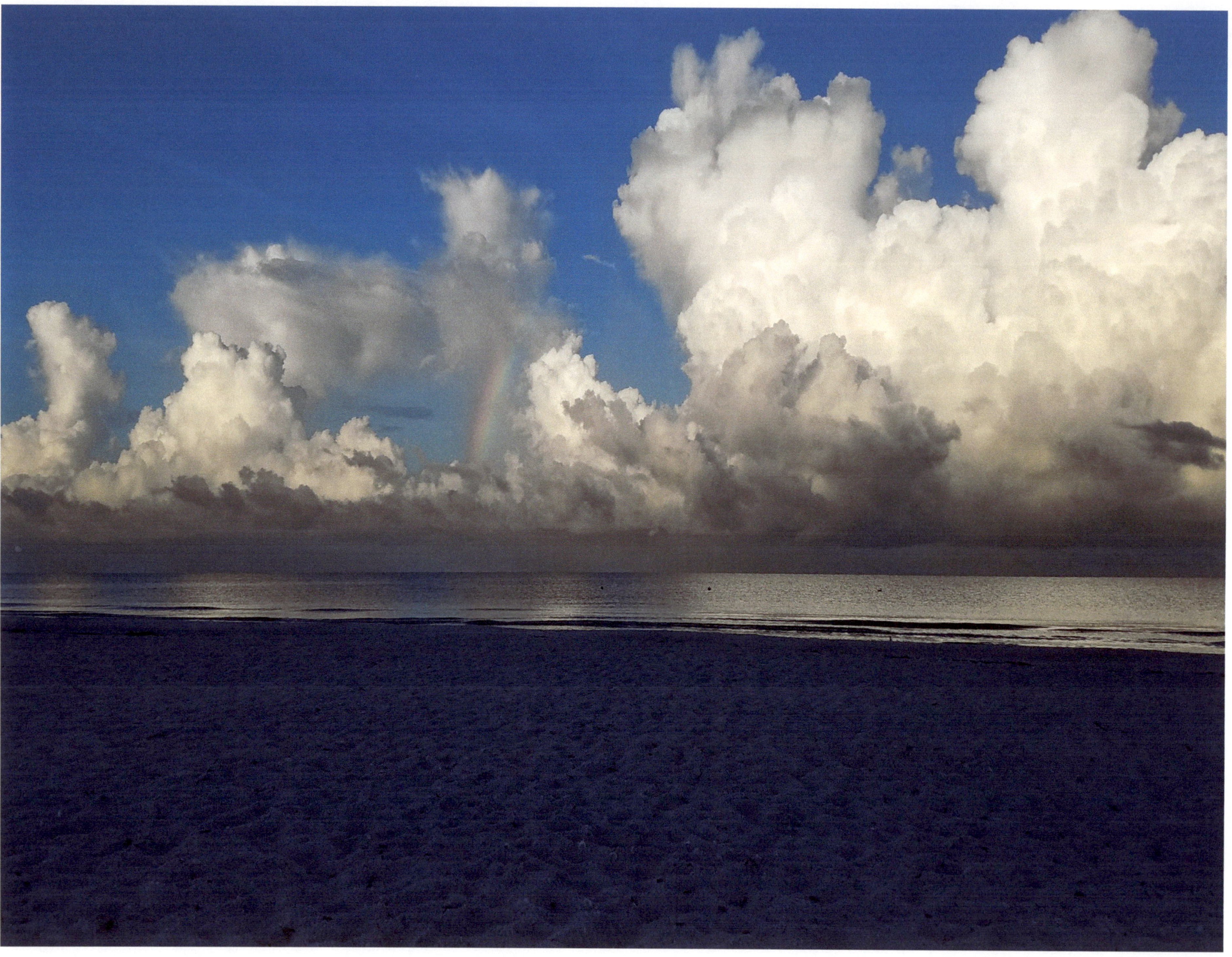

Non-Conceptual

How can your mind be present but not think???? How can your thinking mind be non-conceptual? Aren't all moments thinking moments where you try to work on something, figure something out, or solve some problem?

Well, quite frankly, no they are not.

Look at the photo on the opposite page. What is there to figure out about it? It just IS. It is perfect just the way it is (just like you are).

All your mind needs to do is *notice* it and *accept* it for what it is. It is blue and gray. It is a brilliant rainbow bursting through the clouds. It is a shimmering body of water that stretches to the horizon.

When you are mindful of moments like the one captured by the photo on the opposite page all you need to do is notice and accept it for what it is.

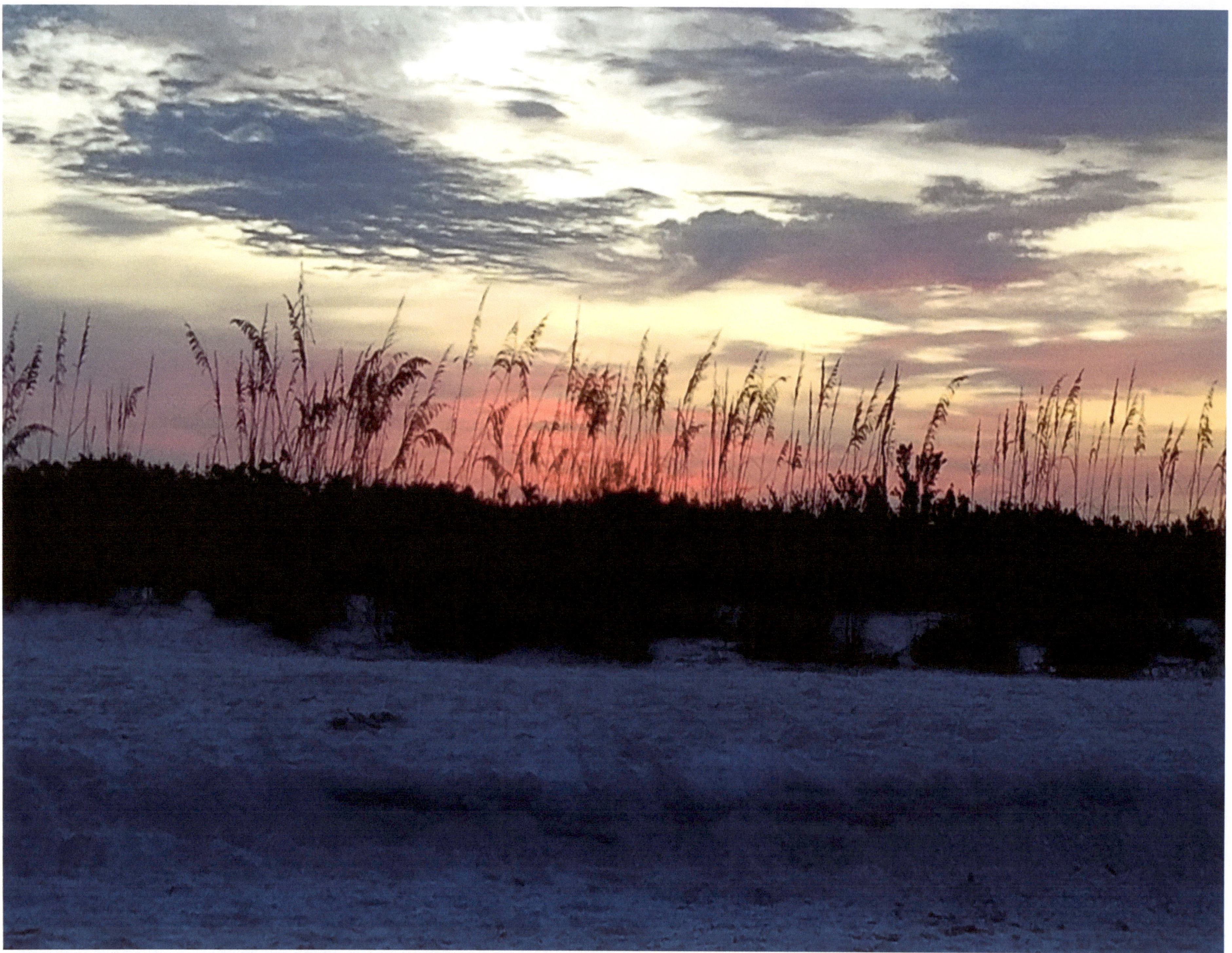

During mindful moments you just notice what is going on in your mind and in your environment. You do not judge what you are experiencing, you accept it for what it is. Accepting reality for what it is, however painful, is a hallmark of mentally healthy people.

When you watch a sunrise like the one on the opposite page you don't compare it to another sunrise. You don't judge it against some arbitrary standard for what sunrises are supposed to be about according to someone else's standards.

You simply notice the blues,pinks and purples and waving sea grass and accept the sunrise for what it is.

Imagine what your life would be like of you could notice and accept people and things for what they are and not feel threatened or stressed by them or feel that you need to change them in any way.

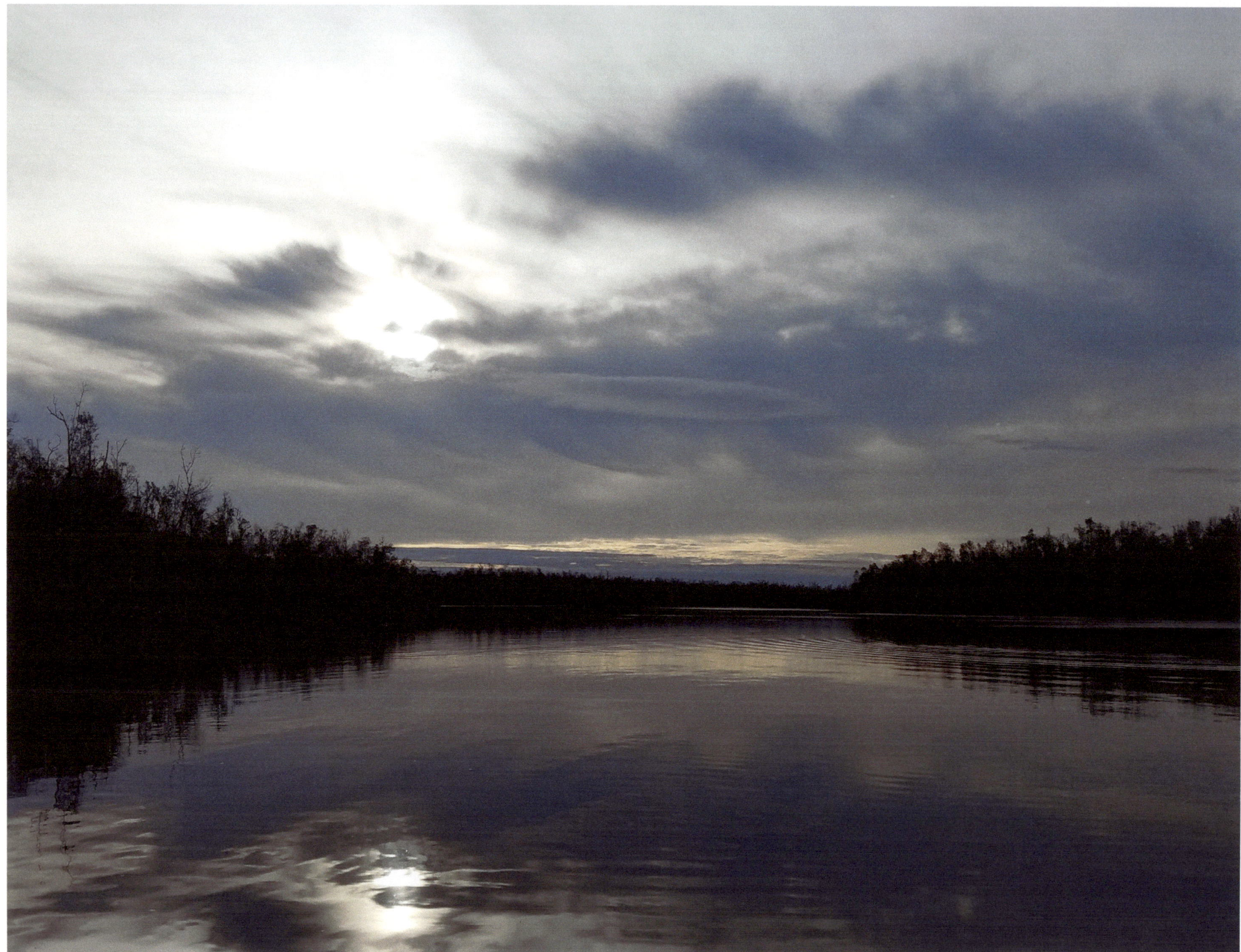

Mindful moments are silent moments. Whenever you add speech to a mindful moment you take it to a conceptual level that takes you *out* of just noticing and *into* thinking about it. The only talking that goes on during mindful moments is self-talk. It is non-verbal and is also known as sub-vocal speech. It should totally revolve around noticing with acceptance.

If you tried to describe the sunrise on the opposite page to another person who was with you it would take you out of being fully present. Invariably you would start thinking and trying to figure out how to describe the image or how it compares to other sunrises. Both of these practices work against being fully mindful and take you out of being 100% focused on the present moment.

Instead, just be quiet and enjoy the beauty that envelopes you.

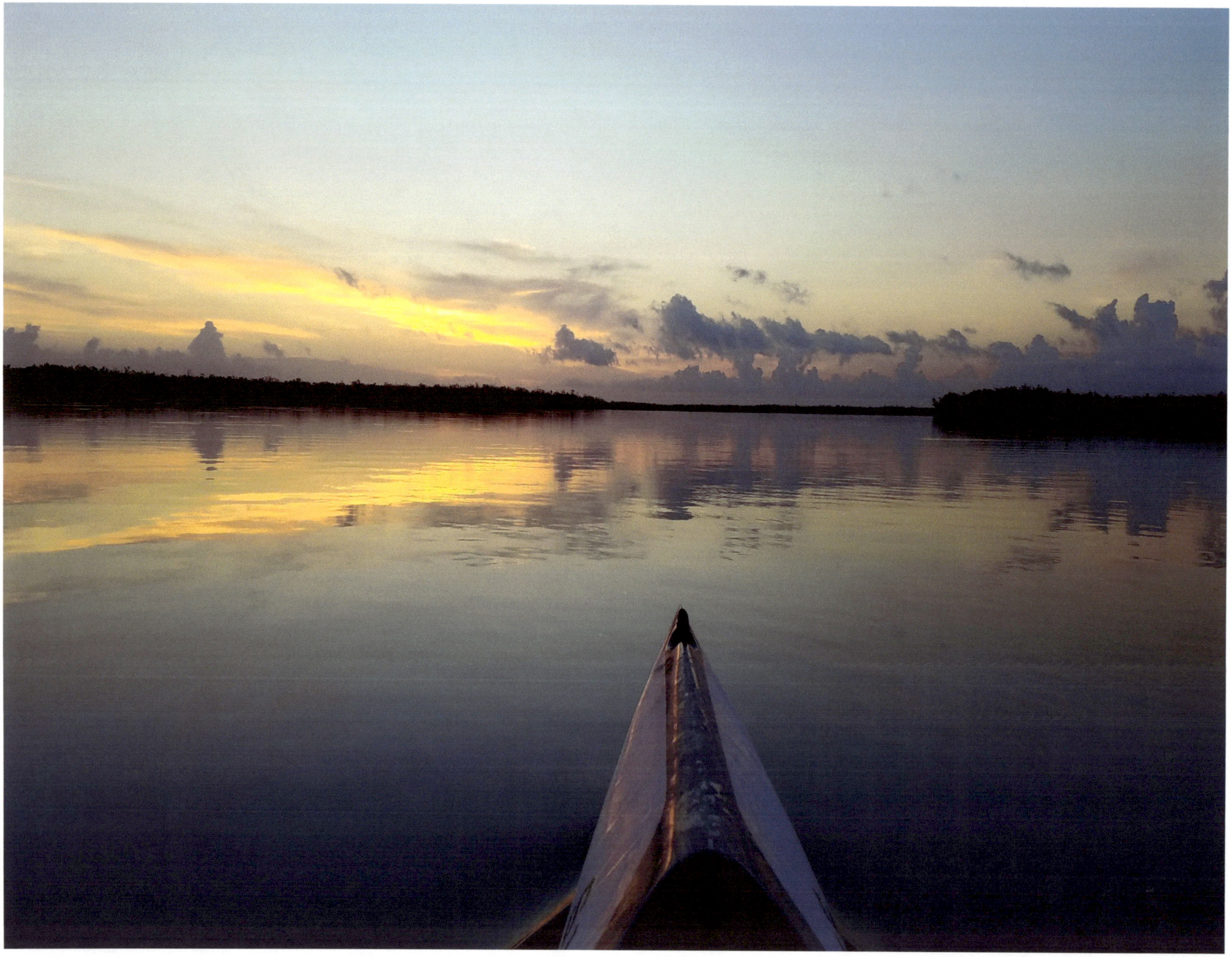

I am a member of a mindfulness meditation group that meets one evening a week on Marco Island. While I love to meditate by myself, I enjoy the fellowship provided by a group of like-minded souls who come together to practice Zazen (just sitting) and share their insights and experiences on their meditation practice.

Those of us who live on Marco Island share in the belief that it is easy to stay in the present moment when we are on the beach or backwaters of our island paradise. Each moment brings a different panorama of clouds, sky, sand, and water. Regardless of how long we have lived here, most of us have not become jaded or take our island paradise for granted. We talk about maintaining our openness to experiencing the island anew each time we venture out to explore her sands and waters.

Buddhists call this state of being the "beginner's mind." Infants and children naturally have a beginner's mind. Take a child to the beach and she will sit in a tide pool and examine a patch of sand and shells for hours. He will sift through the sand, pick out shells and other objects, and smell, touch, and taste them as if they were being experienced for the first time.

As adults we slowly lose our beginner's mind. As we grow up, we get busier and busier. Our hopes, dreams, goals, and plans direct us and we start to lose track of the beauty and bounty around us. We begin to take them for granted as we shift our focus off the present moment and onto acquiring degrees, titles, possessions, and money.

The good news is that we can re-acquire our beginner's mind and shift our focus back onto the present moment by practicing mindfulness. It takes practice to make this mental shift but it is well worth the effort. The practice of mindfulness involves both formal and informal mindfulness training. Formal mindfulness training involves practicing mindfulness meditation on a regular basis. Informal mindfulness training involves practicing simple exercises designed to help you integrate mindfulness into your everyday activities. I call this everyday mindfulness. The rest of this book will focus on formal mindfulness training.

I am going to introduce you to two types of meditation; sitting and moving. As the name implies, sitting meditation is practiced while sitting down. Moving meditation can be performed during any activity that involves continuous motion for at least 20 minutes. I will show you how to perform running and kayaking meditation.

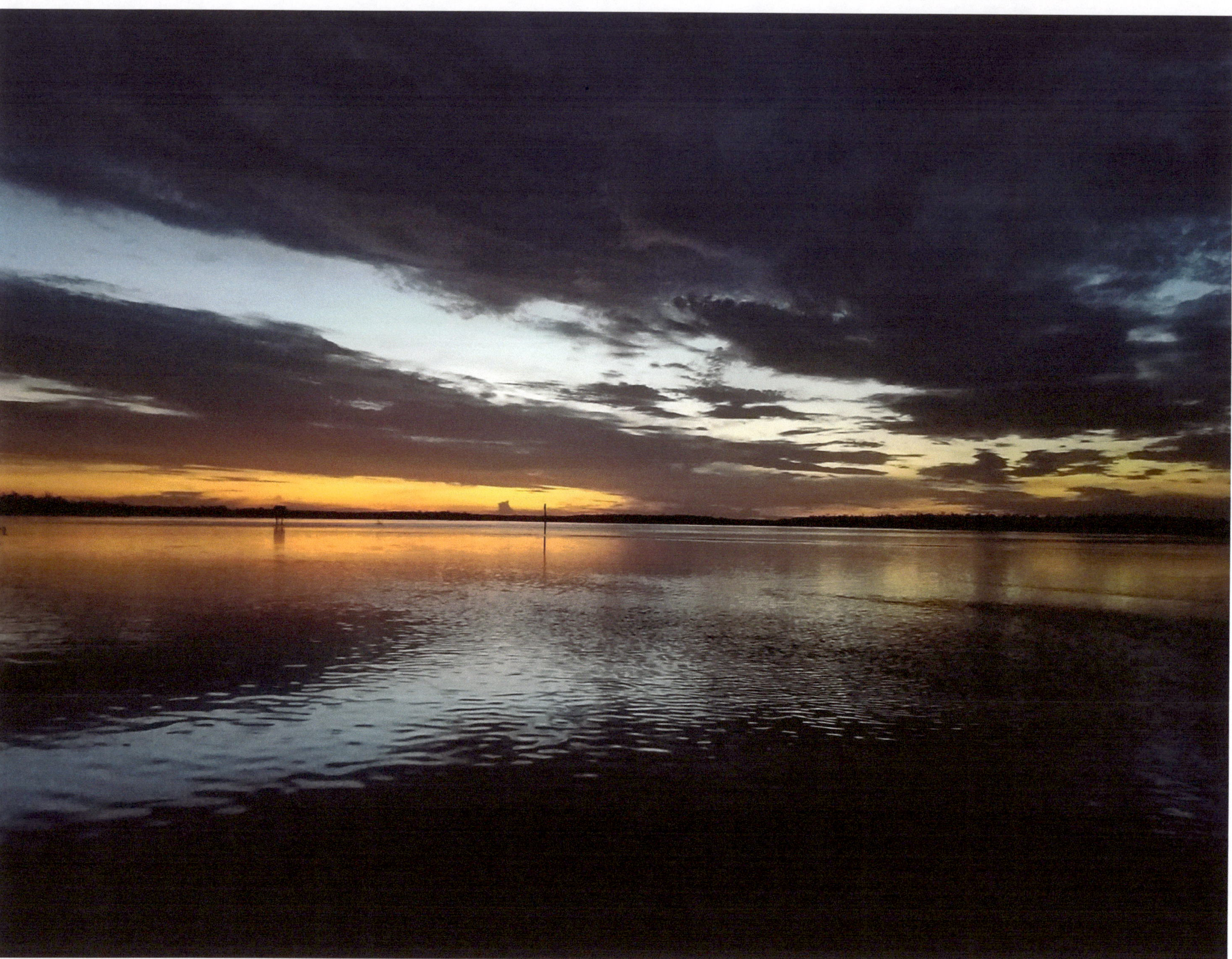

Learning to Meditate

Formal mindfulness training revolves around the regular practice of mindfulness meditation. I ease students and clients into this in three stages:

- diaphragmatic breathing training
- breath meditation training
- mindfulness meditation training

I have found that this approach works because it is incremental in terms of time and focus. For example, you can practice diaphragmatic breathing anywhere, even driving. As little as a few good breaths will help re-direct your focus and make you feel better. To practice either breath meditation or mindfulness meditation you need at least 20 minutes of uninterrupted time and a quiet location free from distractions. Breath meditation uses your breathing as the focal point of your mindfulness. It is more focused and of longer duration than diaphragmatic breathing but easier than mindfulness meditation.

True mindfulness meditation has no single focal point and instead focuses on the endless series of thoughts, feelings, images, and sensations that pass through your mind. It starts with focusing on your breath to get centered but then opens the doors of perception well beyond breathing. For at least 20 minutes you notice the activity of your body, mind, and environment without judgment. When your mind drifts back into the past or jumps into the future you bring your focus back to the present and what is going on in your body, mind, and environment.

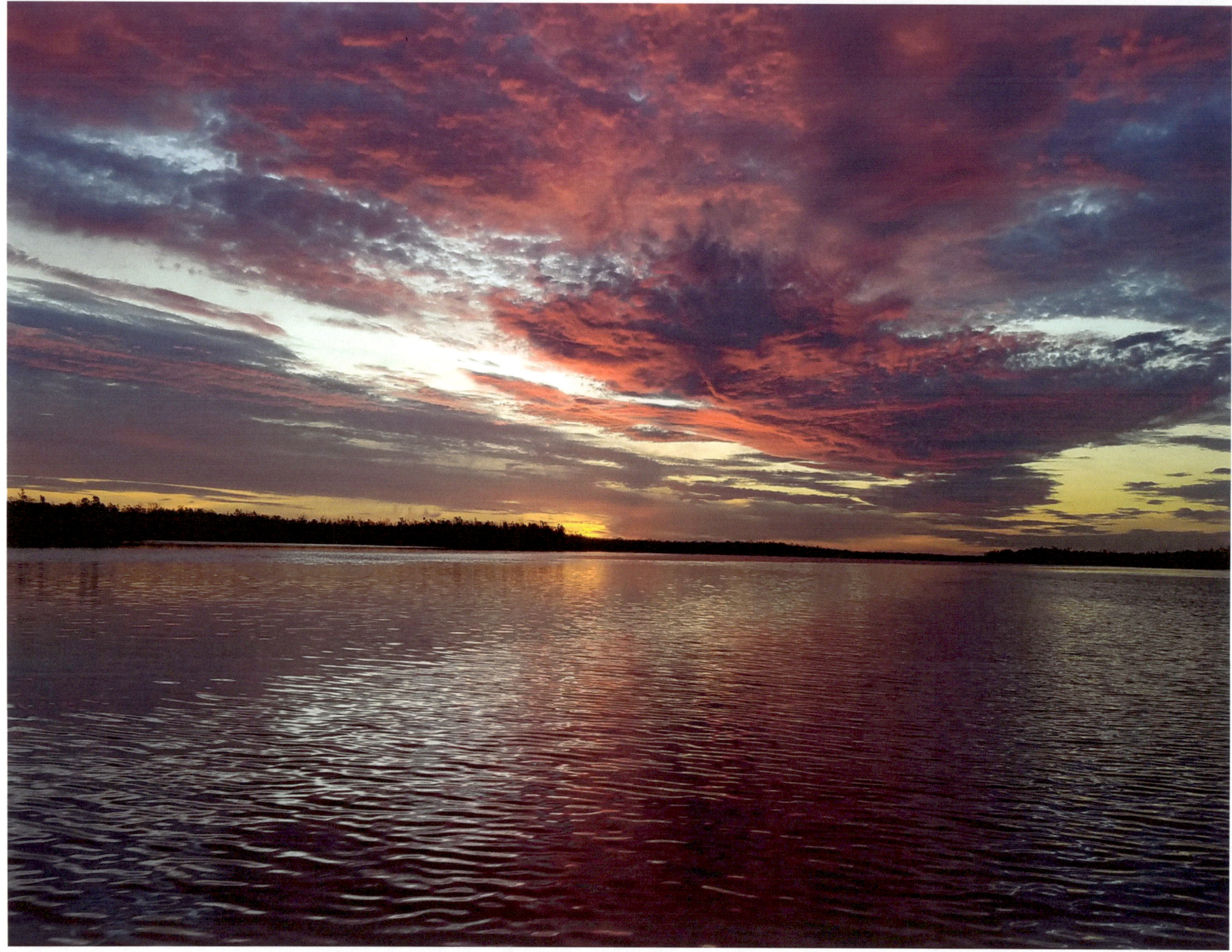

One of the great ironies of breathing is how important it is yet how little attention we pay to it. Although breathing is our biological and spiritual connection to the universe, we usually take it completely for granted. In a sense, every time you breathe you recycle the very elements of life. You breathe in life-giving oxygen and recycle this back into the universe by exhaling carbon dioxide. This cycling of breath in and breath out is your connection to the universe and the cycle of life you share with other living things such as the trees and animals around you. Your breathing is also a spiritual process as this cycle illustrates your interconnectedness to all living things on the planet and the universe beyond.

The simple practice of being more mindful of your breathing can help you get focused and back to the present moment. It can also be used to reduce your stress. When you practice mindful breathing your thinking slows down. Mindful breathing helps you stop over-thinking, especially about past and future worries. The parts of your brain that control breathing are intimately related to the parts that control the stress response. Controlled, deep, even breathing facilitates relaxation. Rapid, shallow, irregular breathing disrupts relaxation. One of the main cues for understanding whether you are stressed is the pace and depth of your breathing. If it is rapid and shallow, chances are that you are stressed.

Most of the time you only use a portion of your lungs when you breathe. You tend to breathe with the top third of your lungs. To receive the calming benefits of diaphragmatic breathing you must learn how to get your entire lungs involved. You need to learn how to fill your lungs completely from the bottom up. Learning how to breathe this way takes practice but you can master it if you spend time each day doing so.

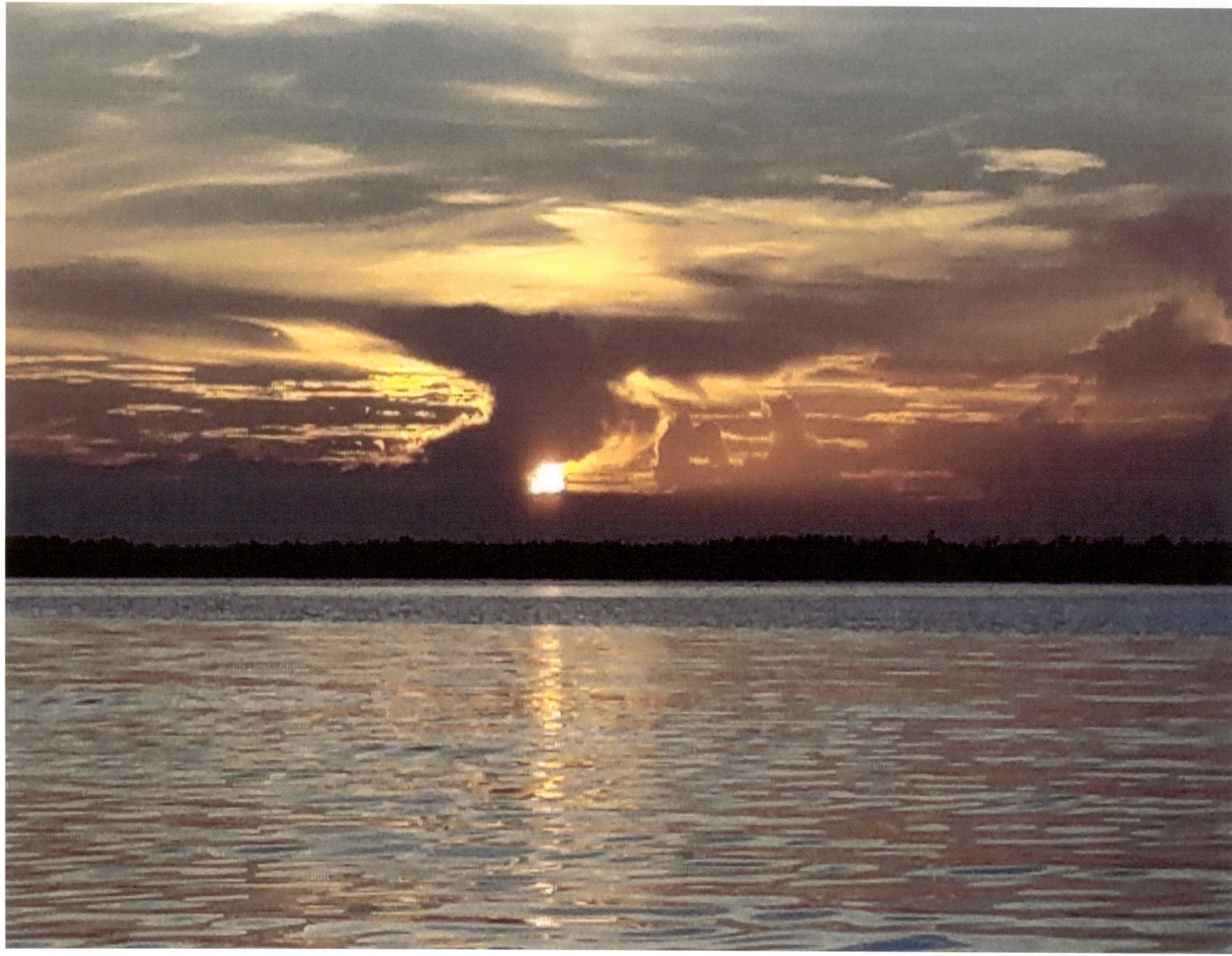

Diaphragmatic Breathing Instructions:

1. Find a relaxing place to sit and gaze out at the scenery (similar to the picture on the opposite page).

2. You can do this in your home if you'd prefer.

3. Focus your attention on your current breathing pattern.

4. Make a mental note of the depth, pace, and regularity of your breathing.

5. Visualize a picture of your lungs and your diaphragm.

6. Slowly breathe in through your nose.

7. Rest your hands on your belly, just under your ribs.

8. Feel your belly move out as your diaphragm pushes down against it.

9. As you breathe in through your nose, visualize your lungs inflating completely starting from the bottom (the part closest to your diiaphragm) and moving upward.

10. Let your ribs expand and shoulders gently rise as your lungs inflate.

11. When you have filled your lungs, slowly exhale through your nose.

12. Feel your belly push back and your diaphragm rise back into place.

13. As you feel the movements in your belly visualize your lungs emptying.

14. Imagine all of the air leaving your lungs as they deflate (sometimes visualizing a balloon losing air or a toothpaste tube squeezing the paste out can be helpful in understanding the emptying process).

15. Continue to breathe in and out this way for a couple of minutes, paying attention to the movement of your belly and diaphragm and the visual picture of your lungs filling from the bottom up and completely emptying.

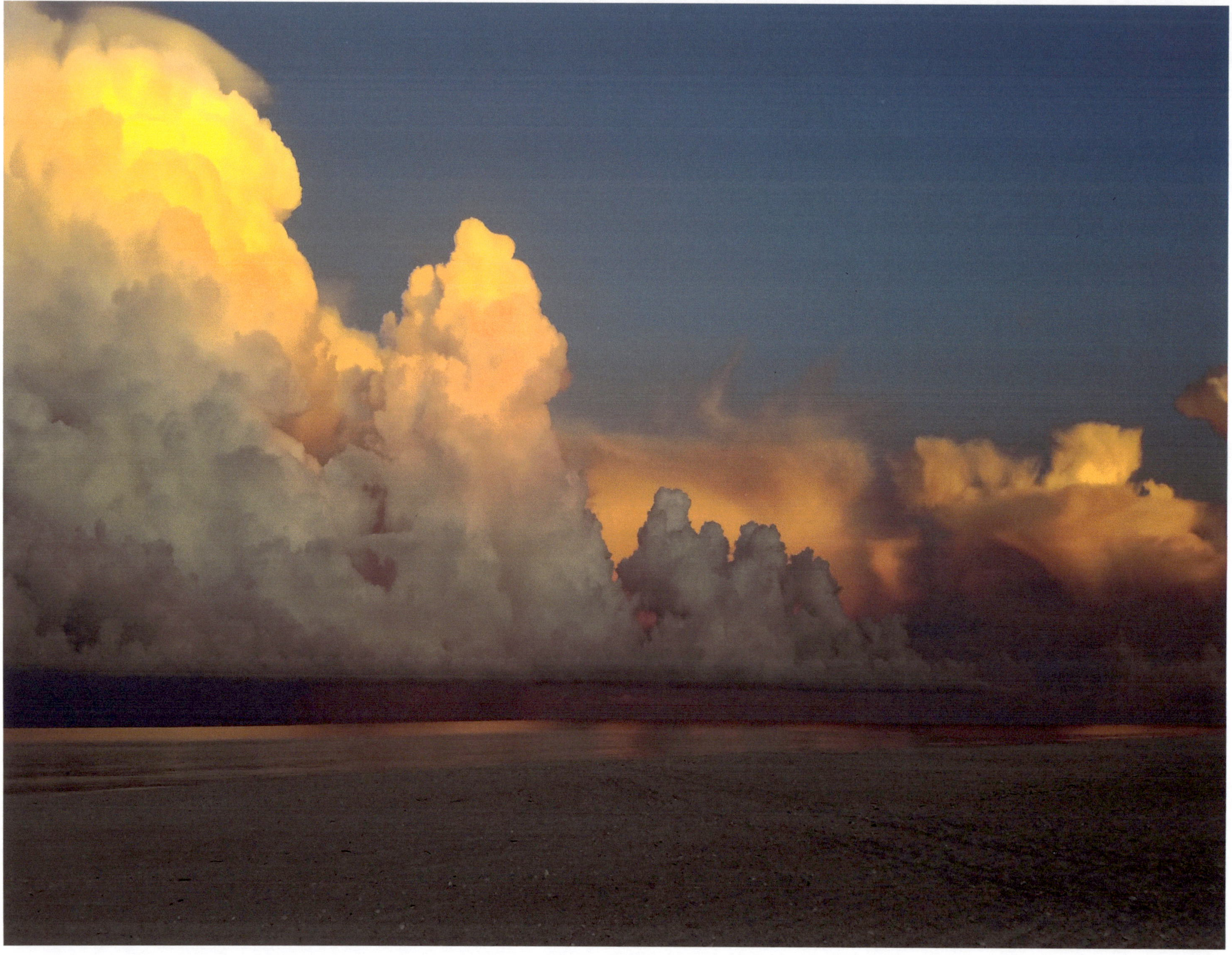

After a week of practicing diaphragmatic breathing I find that most people are comfortable enough with their breathing to use it as a focal point for meditating. When you are able to sit and do diaphragmatic breathing with your eyes open or closed for five minutes you are ready to transform this into a meditative experience.

Three things make breath meditation different from diaphragmatic breathing; focus, intensity, and duration. The focus of breath meditation is the actions of your diaphragm, lungs, and chest as you breathe in and out. While diaphragmatic breathing has a similar focus, it is much less intense.

You can do diaphragmatic breathing with your eyes open while driving, sitting in a meeting, or doing a number of different things. You don't have to give it 100% of your attention. You can't practice Breath Meditation this way. You need to give it 100% of your attention.

I always advise new meditators to do your breath meditation with your eyes closed so you can give it 100% of your attention and minimize distractions. When you do get distracted you simply return your focus to what is going on in your diaphragm, lungs, and chest as you breathe in and out.

The duration of the two practices is also different. A few good diaphragmatic breaths will calm your mind and help you get centered. However, they will *not* give you a meditative effect. To achieve a meditative state, you'll need to sit and meditate for at least 20 undisturbed minutes. It is only after that amount of time that your vital signs (heart rate, respiration, blood pressure) and brain wave activity change.

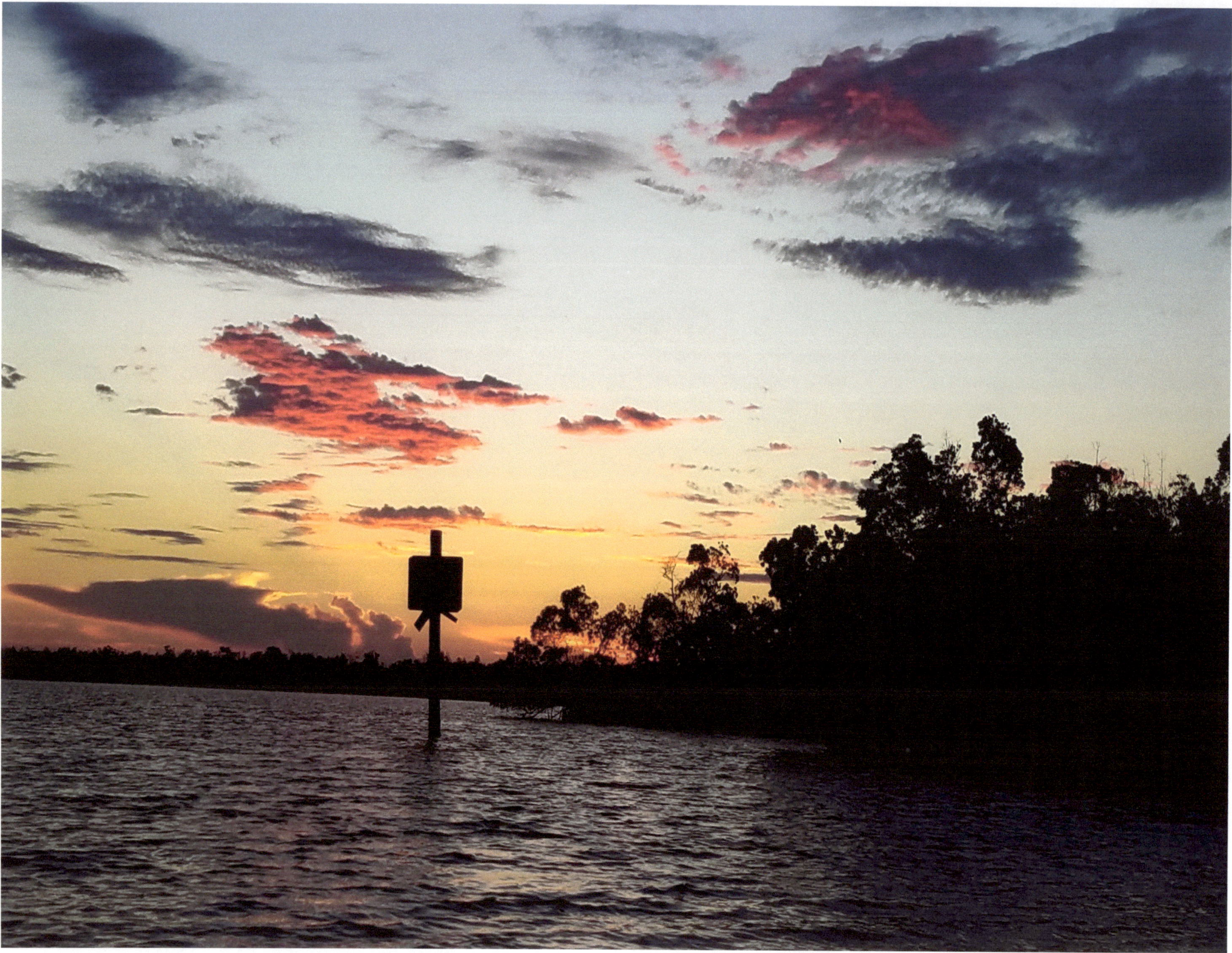

1. Find a relaxing place to sit and gaze out at the scenery (similar to the picture on the opposite page).

2. You can do this in your home if you'd prefer.

3. Set a timer for five minutes. Each week add 1 minute until you can sit and meditate for 20 uninterrupted minutes.

4. Sit quietly in a chair, with your feet flat on the floor, back straight, and hands folded gently in your lap.

5. Focus your attention on your current breathing pattern. Make a mental note of the depth, pace, and regularity of your breathing.

6. Visualize a picture of your lungs and your diaphragm and slowly breathe in through your nose and feel your belly move out as your diaphragm pushes down against it.

7. Let your ribs expand and shoulders gently rise as your lungs inflate.

8. When you have filled your lungs, slowly exhale through your nose. Feel your belly push back and your diaphragm rise back into place.

9. Your mind will wander throughout your session. This is normal and still happens to veteran meditators. You might find that saying "in" as you inhale and "out" as you exhale makes it easier to keep your focus on your breathing. Say these words to yourself. Some people find that counting the seconds it takes to inhale and exhale keeps them focused on their breathing.

10. When your thoughts stray from the present moment do not get upset at yourself. Instead, tell yourself: "My mind is taking me out of the here and now" and then get back to focusing on your breathing.

11. Continue meditating until your timer goes off.

12. Practice at least three times a week, slowly increasing your time from 5-20 minutes.

     With a few months practice, you will find that you can slow your breathing down and stay focused on it most of the time. Be patient and forgiving with yourself as you practice breath meditation. It will take time and practice to get comfortable with it, but it is time well spent.

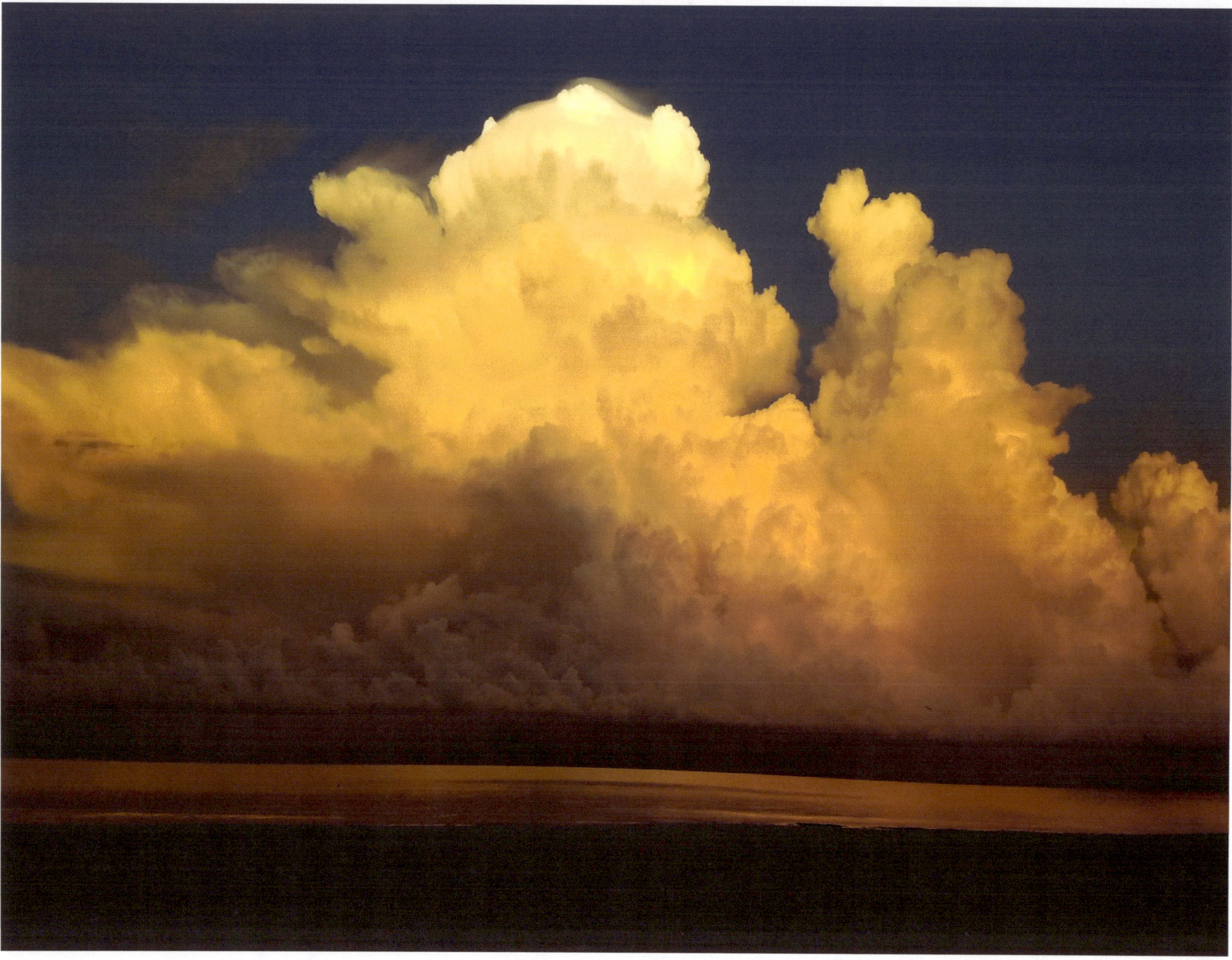

Mindfulness Meditation

Mindfulness meditation is often referred to as "Just Sitting." The just sitting reference is both very descriptive and very misleading. In one sense, all you do when you perform mindfulness meditation is "just sit" for an extended period of time. This sounds pretty simple, direct, and uncomplicated. However, unlike other times when you just sit, during mindfulness meditation you not only sit, you also pay full attention to **everything** going on inside and outside your body and mind, as well as in the environment around you. In other words, you're fully aware of all your thoughts, self-talk, mental images, and emotions. You're also fully aware of the sensations going on in your body. These might be related to muscle tension, pain, breathing, or any other physiologic activities than you sense. In addition, you're aware of things going on around you. You're aware of the temperature and movement of air, sounds, scents, and anything else emanating from your environment. Your experience is 100 percent focused on the here and now and your internal and external environments. Unlike Breath Meditation, which is designed to relax your body and mind, Mindfulness Meditation is designed to increase your awareness of what is going on in your internal and external environments.

Mindfulness Meditation uses your breath as a focal point but only when your mind wanders out of the present moment and into the past or future. It also uses your breath as a tool to return to the present moment when you become aware that your mind is judging, comparing, problem solving or doing something other than just noticing and accepting. During Mindfulness Meditation there is no attempt to censor your incoming thoughts, sounds, and other stimuli as long as they are related to the present.

Many people are frustrated when they initially learn how to perform mindfulness meditation because their focus is constantly interrupted by competing thoughts, feelings, and external stimuli. When they become aware of these distractions they react emotionally, becoming upset with themselves for allowing the distraction. Rather than ignoring, suppressing, or evaluating these disruptions and thus getting emotionally involved with them, it is better to just note their presence, accept them, and continue to meditate. A key to understanding mindfulness meditation is realizing that it is based on developing an accepting attitude toward reality. The idea is to observe reality in a noncritical way.

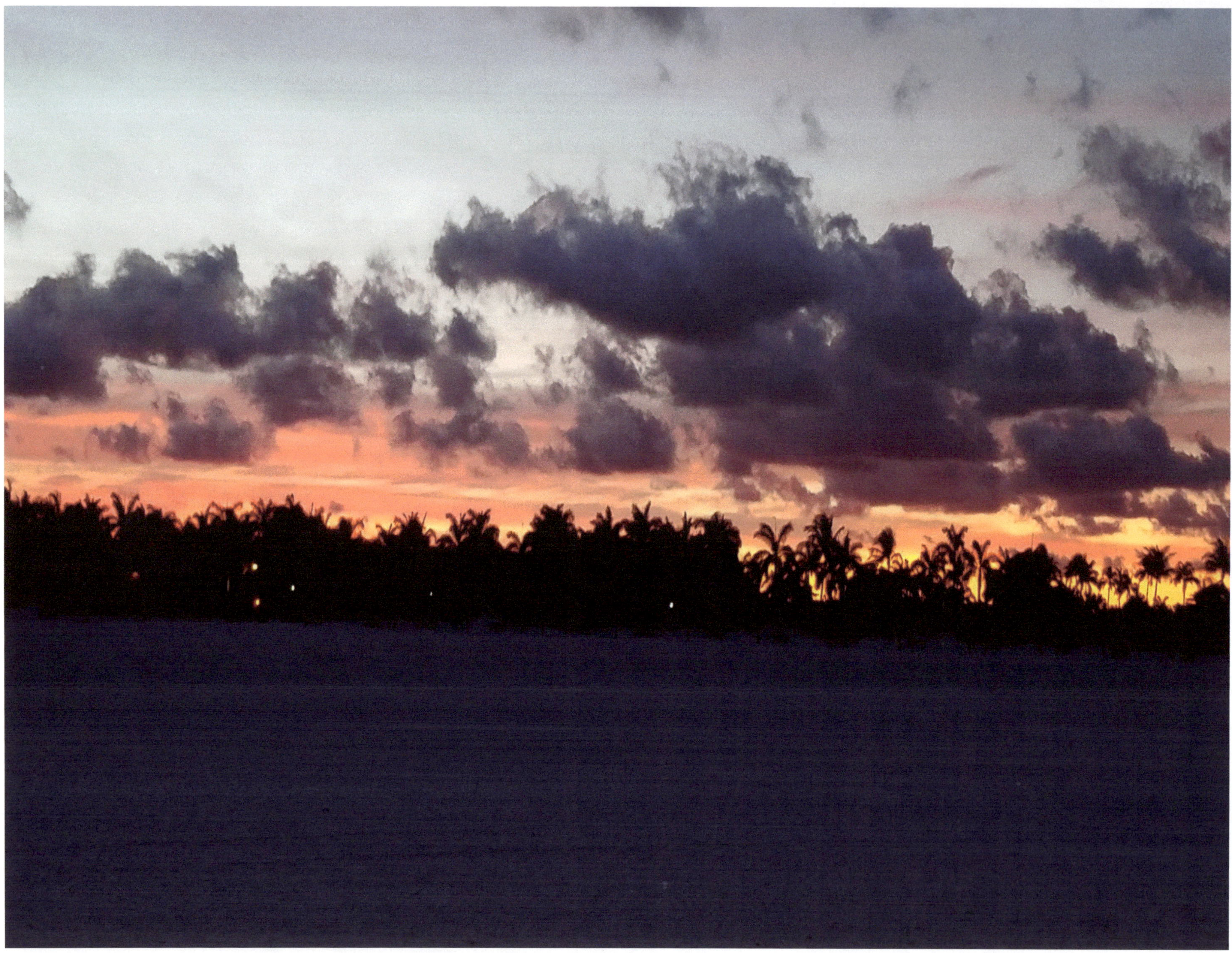

Mindfulness Meditation Instructions:

1. Find a relaxing place to sit and gaze out at the scenery (similar to the picture on the opposite page). You can do this in your home if you'd prefer.

2. Set a timer for five minutes. Each week add 1 minute until you can sit and meditate for 20 uninterrupted minutes.

3. Sit quietly in a chair, with your feet flat on the floor, back straight, and hands folded gently in your lap.

4. Focus your attention on your breathing. Do not attempt to regulate or control your breathing (like you do in breath meditation). Simply close your eyes and notice the depth, pace, and regularity of your breathing for several breaths.

5. Notice the sensations in your chest, abdomen, shoulders and neck as you breathe in and out. Feel your chest muscles expand and contract and your shoulders rise and fall as you breathe. Notice what happens in your neck and head as you breathe in and out.

6. Continue to breathe for several more breaths and then shift your focus to the rest of your body. Notice the sensations in the rest of your body as you breathe in and out.

7. Focus your attention on something on the near or far horizon. Notice the color, shape, size, patterns, etc. of the object(s) in your visual field. Do not judge or compare what you are seeing or try to figure out why they look the way they do, just accept them.

8. As you gaze out on your focal point pay attention to the sounds in your immediate environment. Don't try to figure out anything about them, just enjoy the sounds for what they are.

9. Shift your focus to the other sensations in your environment. Notice the temperature and feelings of warmth or coldness as they waft over your body. Notice the volume, direction, and intensity of air flowing around you. Notice any smells that enter your mind.

10. Continue to breathe normally as you focus on the horizon and notice the things going in your body, mind, and environment.

11. Your mind will wander throughout your session. When your thoughts stray from the present moment do not get upset at yourself. Instead, tell yourself: "There goes my mind again taking me out of the present moment" and then shift your focus onto your breathing.

12. Open your eyes and continue meditating until your timer goes off. Practice at least three times a week, slowly increasing your time from 5-20 minutes. With a few months practice you will find that you can stay focused on the present moment most of the time.

     Be patient and forgiving with yourself as you practice mindfulness meditation. It will take time and practice to get comfortable with it, but it is time well spent.

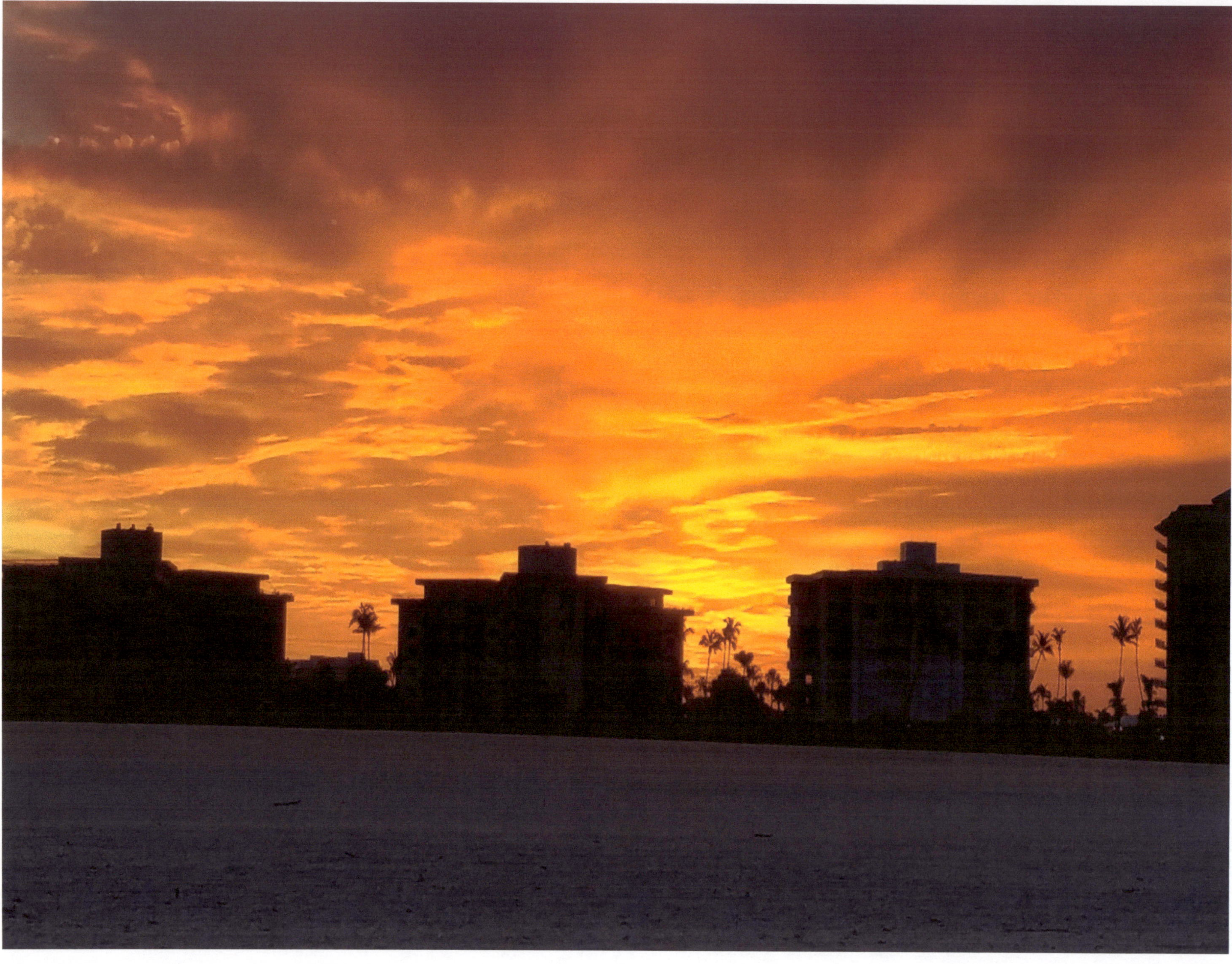

Getting Distracted and Re-Focused

When you meditate you will get distracted. It is just the nature of your mind to do so. Your mind is a lot like your computer. If you leave your computer on its programs will run non-stop, 24/7 processing information. Your mind also has programs that run non-stop, 24/7. Your mind's programs are your thoughts, feelings, self-talk, and mental images. These programs constantly run and make it very easy for you to get distracted and taken out of being in the present moment.

When you get distracted because of the non-stop nature of your mind it is usually because it:

- jumps out of the present moment to the past or the future
- runs away with non-stop thinking and problem solving
- judges, evaluates, and compares instead of just noticing and accepting

It doesn't matter what type of meditation you are practicing (sitting or moving), you're going to get distracted and have to get your mind back to the present moment. The following four steps will help you return your focus to the present moment:

- Notice that you are distracted
- Accept that it happened
- Be forgiving
- Redirect your focus to your breathing

When you get distracted simply say to yourself; "There goes my runaway mind again taking me out of the present moment. It is OK, I am only human." Then redirect your focus to whatever your original focal point was (clouds, water, paddling etc.). Be patient and forgiving, it will take a while to get comfortable with meditating. Enjoy the journey.

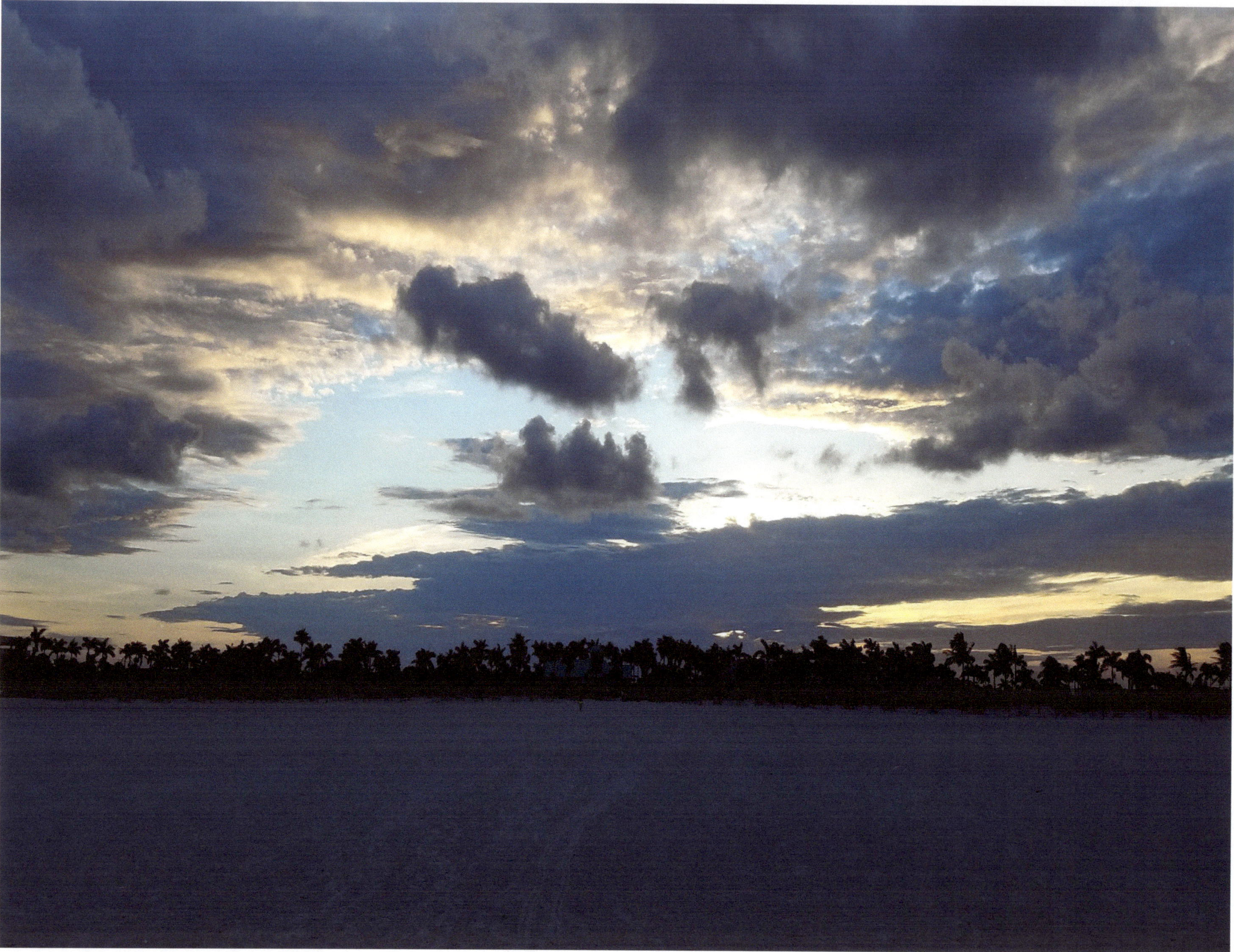

Cloud meditation is a form of focused meditation (like breath meditation). All form of focused meditation use some object as a focal point. Examples of common focal points used in meditation are your breath, a mantra (secret word), candle flame, mandala, or crystal.

One of the most amazing things about Marco Island is its' constantly shifting pattern of clouds that come and go. They make it easy to sit and meditate because their majesty is mesmerizing.

Look at the sheer size of the cloud on the opposite page and imagine sitting on the beach as it envelopes you. Besides it's towering size, the colors of the morning reflect on it and provide a minute-by-minute changing kaleidoscope of colors and shapes.

Since cloud meditation is a specific form of sitting meditation, you follow the general guidelines for Breath Meditation but use a cloud or cloud formation as your focal point.

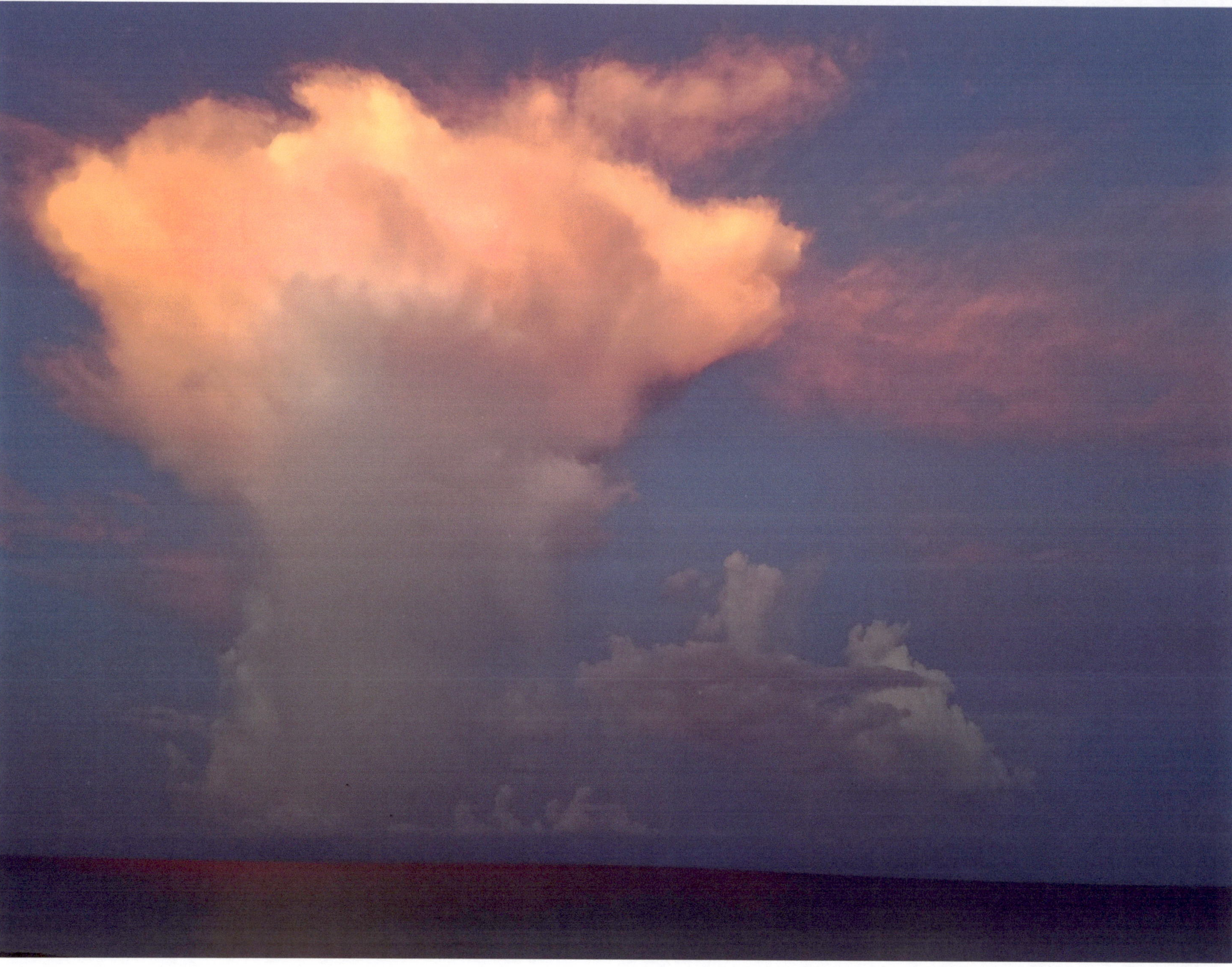

Cloud Meditation Instructions

1. Find a relaxing place to sit and gaze out at the clouds where you won't be disturbed by others.

2. Set a timer for five minutes. Each week add 1 minute until you can sit and meditate for 20 uninterrupted minutes.

3. Sit quietly in a chair, with your feet flat on the floor, back straight, and hands folded gently in your lap.

4. Focus your attention on your current breathing pattern. Make a mental note of the depth, pace, and regularity of your breathing.

5. Slowly breathe in through your nose and feel your belly move out as your diaphragm pushes down against it.

6. When you have filled your lungs, slowly exhale through your nose, feeling your diaphragm rise back into place.

7. Pick one specific area and focus your attention on the clouds in the sky.

8. Notice their size, shape, color, and movement as the wind affects the.

9. Say the word "clouds" to yourself as you inhale and exhale.

10. When your thoughts stray from the present moment do not get upset at yourself. Instead, tell yourself: "My mind is taking me out of the here and now" and then get back to focusing on the word clouds as you slowly breathe in and out.

11. Continue meditating until your timer goes off.

12. Practice at least three times a week, slowly increasing your time from 5-20 minutes.

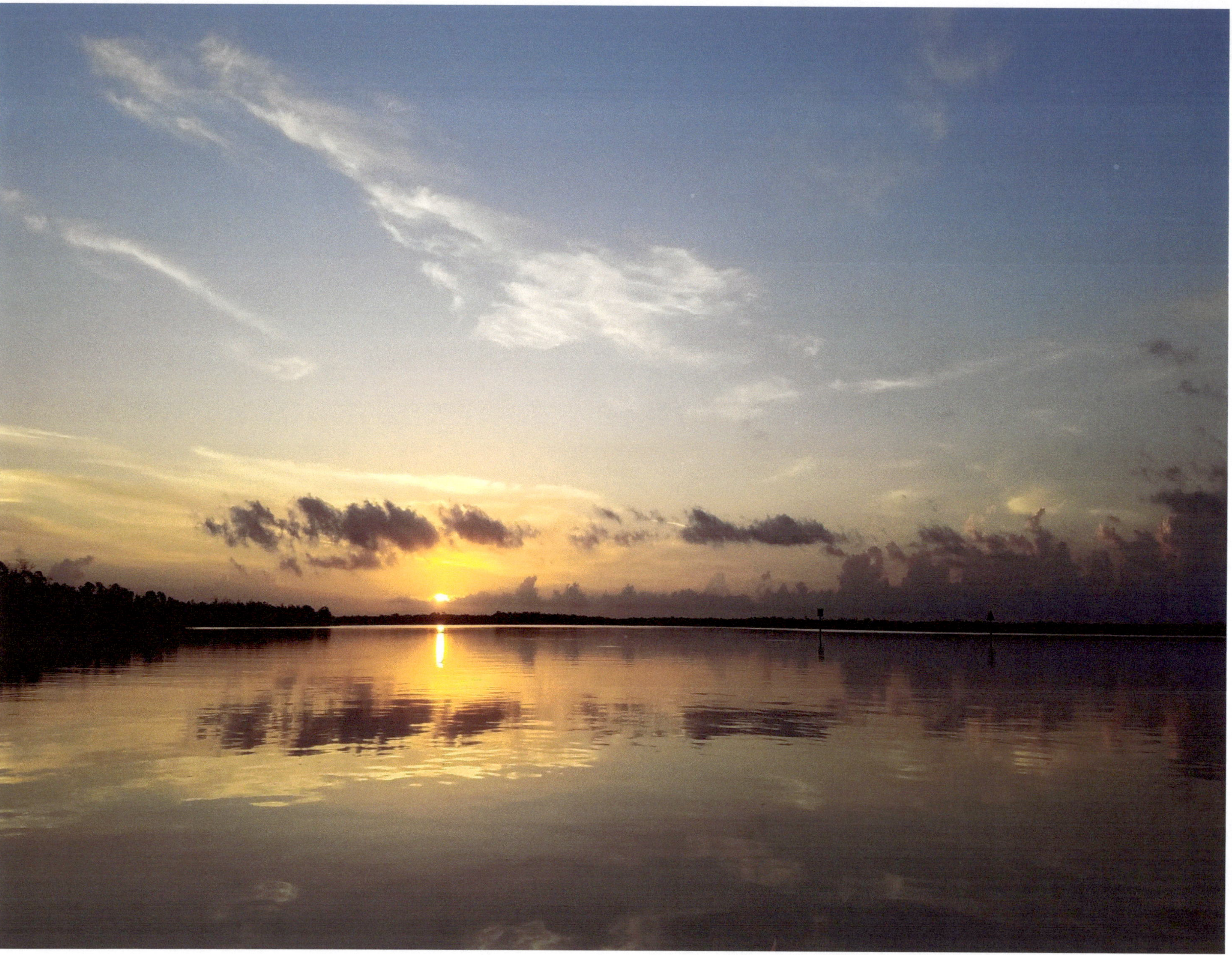

Many people tell me that they'd love to learn how to meditate and practice mindfulness, but they can't sit still long enough to learn. The thought of sitting quietly in the same place for 10, 20, or 30 minutes stresses them out just thinking about it. They'd rather walk, run, bike, or swim to deal with their stress and nervous energy.

If that sounds like you, then moving meditation is right up your alley. Unlike traditional meditation, which is practiced while sitting quietly, moving meditation uses the movements that accompany any repetitive continuous physical activity as the focal point.

Walking, running, swimming, bicycling, and cross-country skiing are examples of repetitive, continuous physical activity that typically is sustained for at least twenty minutes and can provide an aerobic training effect as well as a meditative benefit.

My two favorite forms of moving meditation involve running and kayaking because they are done on my two favorite places on Marco Island; the beach and the backwaters of the 10,000 islands.

I'll show you how you can get both a meditative and aerobic (if you wish) effect while engaging in these two activities.

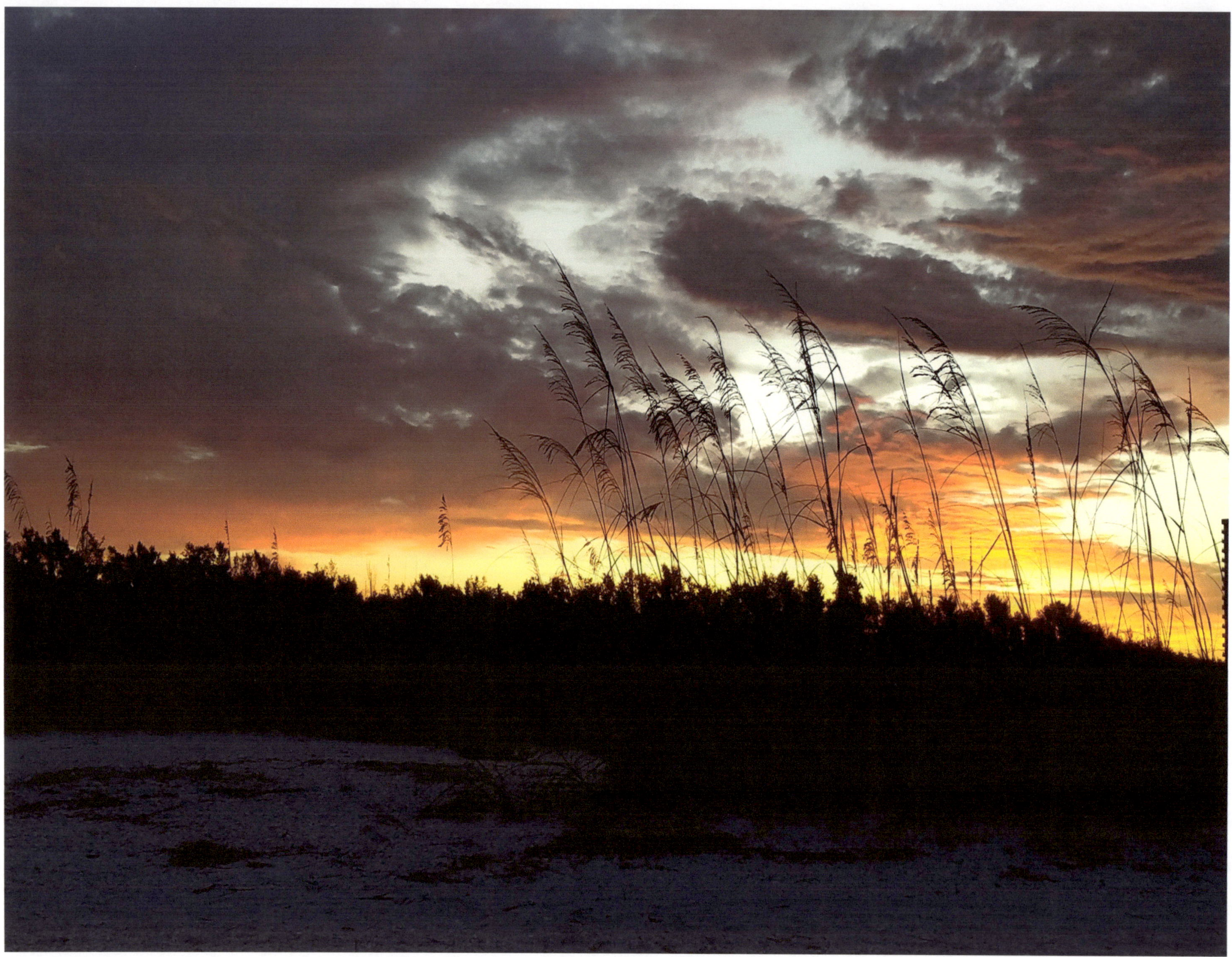

Walking/Running Meditation

Walking is an excellent activity to use to learn moving meditation because it is safe, can be practiced by almost anyone, and can be done both indoors on a treadmill and outdoors. It also is an excellent starting point for those who ultimately want to begin a running program.

During walking meditation, you use the individual components of each step (lifting the leg, bending the knee, stepping forward, heel touching, toe touching, etc.), as your focal point. You also pay attention to the *process* of walking (feelings in the feet, legs, back, etc., one's balance and sensation of movement), and your breathing.

You can also synchronize your footfalls and your breathing pattern to help you minimize distracting thoughts while you focus on what is going on in your legs, feet, and hips as you walk. To do this you first need to determine how many steps you take with each inhalation and exhalation. For example, I take six steps with each inhalation and six steps with each exhalation when I am walking. When I am running, I take three breaths with every inhalation and three with every exhalation. Once you know how many steps you take to fill and empty your lungs, you simply count "one, two, three, four" in synchrony with each step as you inhale and exhale. Synchronizing like this will help you focus on your breathing and footfalls rather than the thousand and one other things running around your brain when you walk or run.

The major difference between walking and running meditation is the intensity. If you want to achieve both an aerobic and meditative effect, you have to walk or run at a speed that elevates your heart rate into your aerobic training zone* and keep it there for at least 20 minutes. Most walkers do not intentionally walk at such a pace.

* Your Aerobic Training Zone is between 65% - 85% of your Maximum Attainable Heart Rate (MHR). To find this zone subtract your age from 220 and multiply that number by .65 and .85. The resulting numbers give you the low and high end of your training zone. As long as you keep your heart rate in that zone for 20 minutes you will get an aerobic workout.

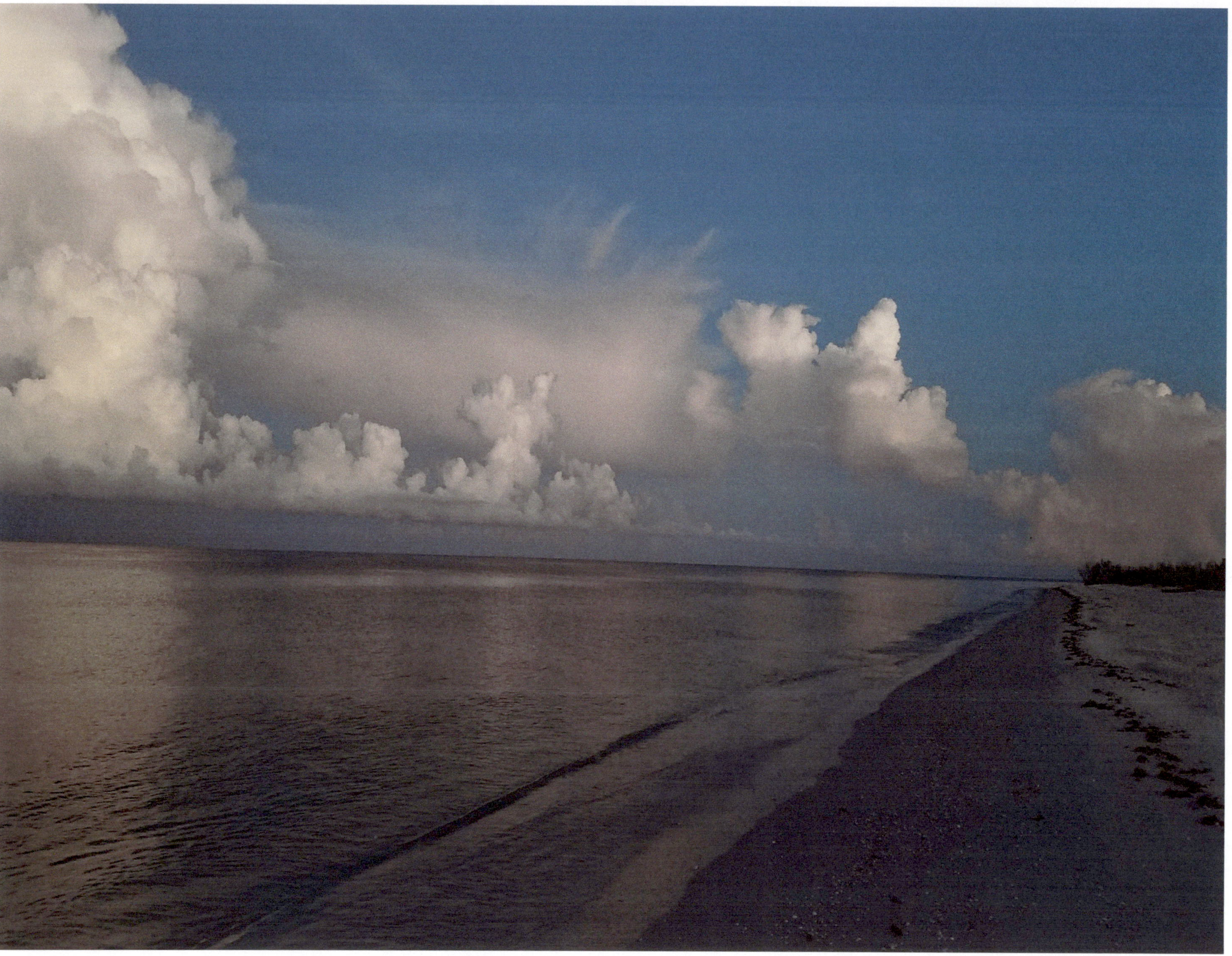

Instructions for Walking/Running Meditation:

1. I recommend walking or running on the beach on the hard-packed sand close to the waterline.

2. Warm up by walking at a slow-moderate pace for 5 minutes.

3. If you want to get an aerobic training effect, increase your pace and get into your Aerobic Training Zone. *If you just want to do walking meditation walk at a comfortable brisk pace.

4. Pay attention to your breathing (inhalation and exhalation) for a couple of minutes.

5. Count (to yourself) the number of steps it takes to fully inflate your lungs.

6. Count (to yourself) the number of steps it takes to fully deflate your lungs.

7. For the next several minutes focus on synching your walking/running pace with your inhalations and exhalations.

8. Whenever your mind strays to the future or the past say to yourself, "there goes my mind again taking me out of the present moment" and refocus on counting your steps and synching them to your breathing.

9. Shift your attention to your feet, legs, knees, and hips as you continue to walk.

10. Pay attention to each footfall (striking with the heel of your foot, rolling forward onto the ball and forefoot, pushing off gently with your toes)

12. Pay attention to your footfalls for several steps.

13. Shift your focus to your ankles and lower legs as you continue to walk.

14. Notice how your ankles and lower legs contract and relax in relation to each footfall.

15. Pay attention to your ankles and lower legs for several steps.

16. Shift your focus to your knees and upper legs as you continue to walk.

17. Notice how your knees and upper legs contract and relax in relation to each footfall.

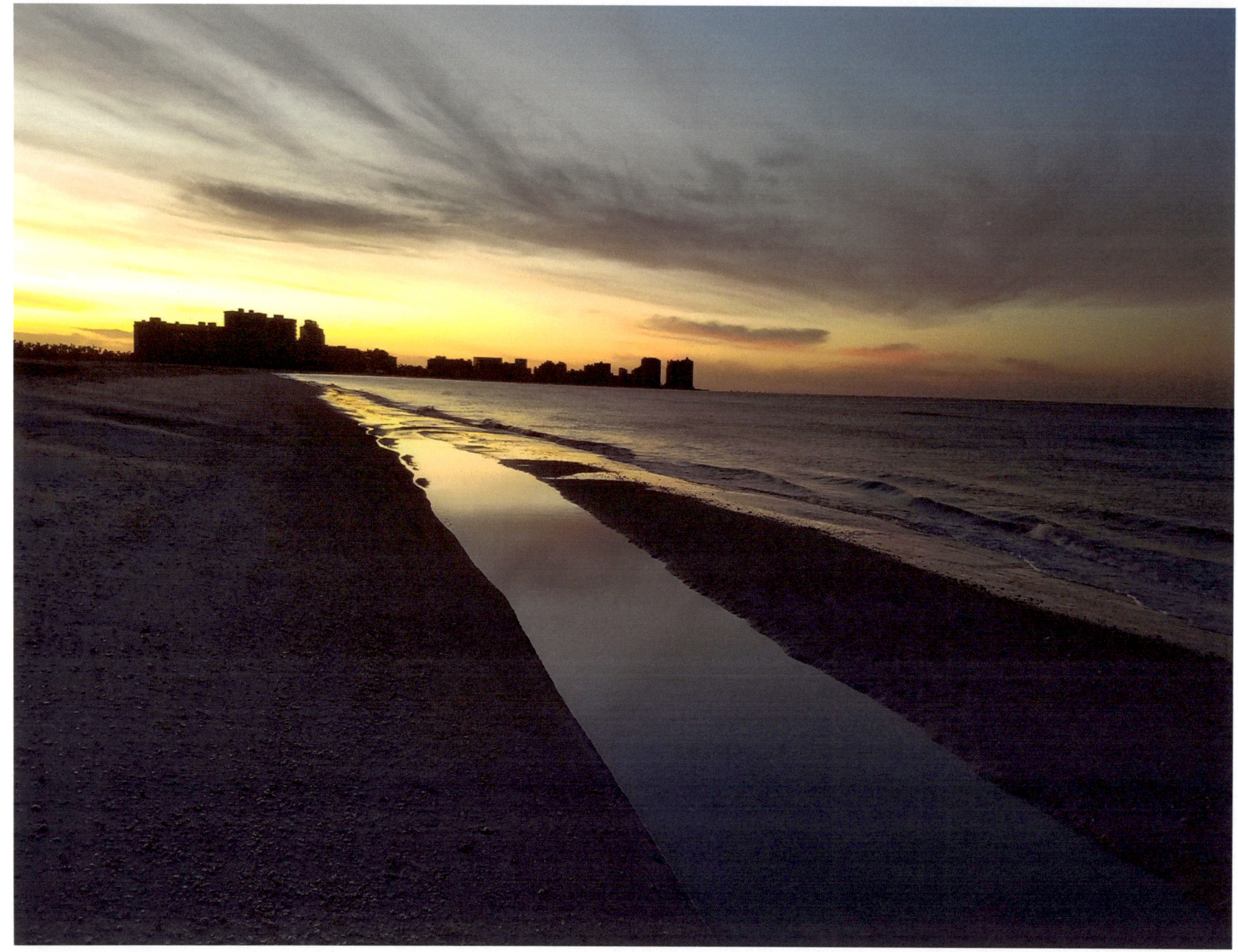

18. Pay attention to your knees and upper legs for several steps.

19. Shift your focus to your hips as you continue to walk.

20. Notice how your hips sway in relation to each step.

21. Feel your hip muscles contract and relax in relation to each footfall.

22. Pay attention to your hips for several steps.

23. Shift your focus to the complete walking process from footfall through hip contraction and flexion.

24. Focus on the fluid nature of your gait as you walk or run effortlessly on the sand, breathing deeply and steadily and counting off your cadence to yourself.

25. Do not be critical of yourself if your mind wanders or if you have a difficult time focusing on your muscles. Simply note what is going on and get back to your breathing and observation of your walking or running.

26. Continue walking this way for 20–30 minutes.

27. At the end of your time cool down for five minutes by walking at a slow-moderate pace for 5 minutes.

The picture on the opposite page is a typical scene for my sunrise running meditation sessions on Marco Island.

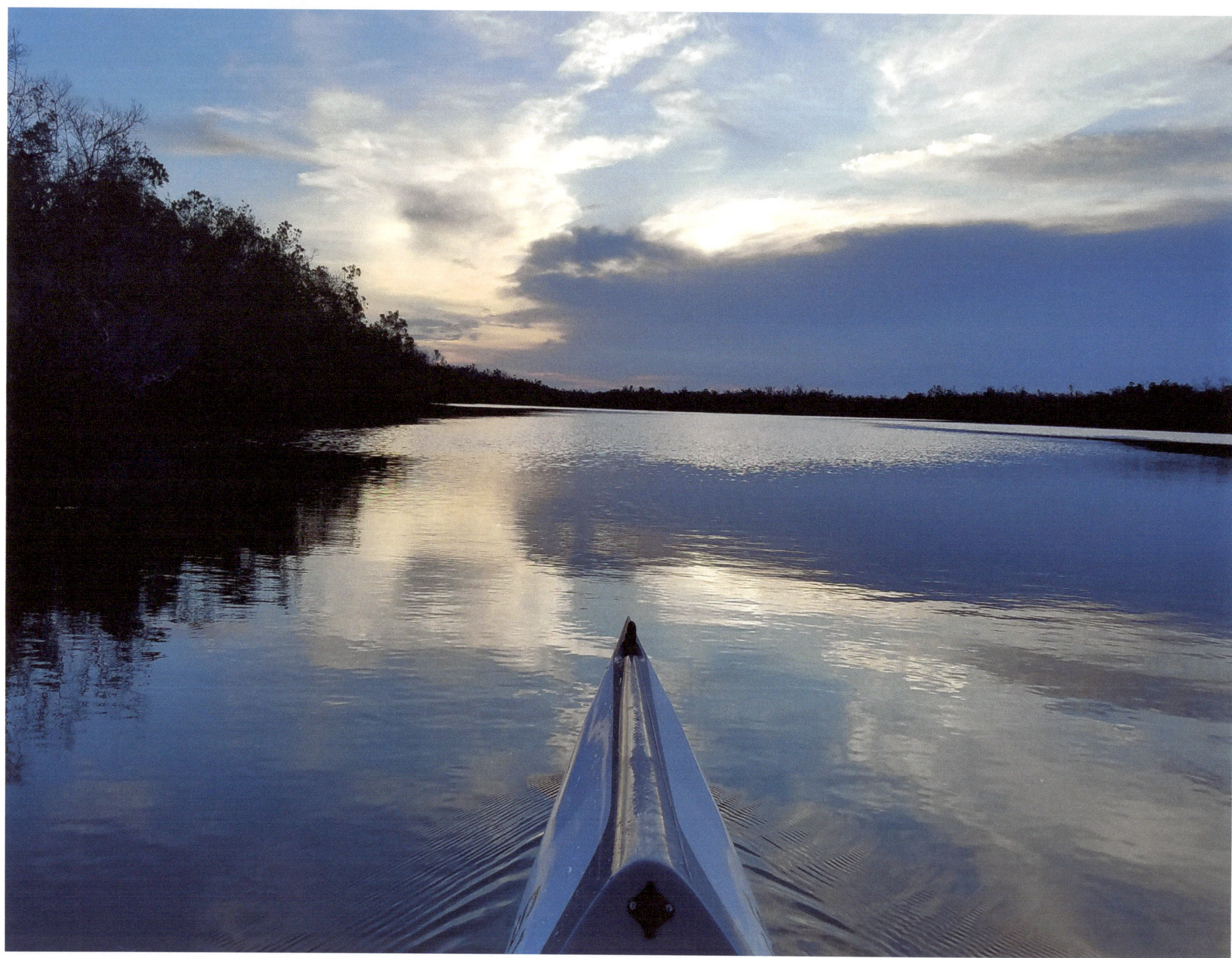

Kayak Meditation

Sometimes I turn my sunrise kayaking outings into moving meditations. The peace and serenity of being on the water as the sun rises is unmatched. If you paddle by yourself as I do when I do kayak meditation the silence is only broken by natural sounds or the ripples from my paddle or boat gently moving through the water. Some of the natural sounds I encounter are birds, the wind, and waves breaking in the mangroves. I feel truly blessed to be able to experience such wonders.

As a form of moving meditation, kayaking meditation is similar to walking/running meditation. Instead of focusing your attention on each footfall, extension, bend of the knee, etc. as you would while walking or running, you focus on your paddle strokes. This involves being fully aware of what is going on in your arms, shoulders, hips, and legs as you dip your paddle into the water, pull it back, twist your torso and hips, and push off with your foot to drive the stroke through the water.

When you perform paddling meditation, you get just as distracted as you would when walking or running. It is easy to get distracted by the sights, sounds, and smells of Marco Island's incredible waterways. When this happens, your mind jumps into the future or back to the past and you find yourself out of the present moment. To minimize this, you focus on synching the cadence of your paddle strokes to your breathing pattern. This is the same technique you used during walking/running meditation when you synched the cadence of your steps to your breathing.

If you are interested in getting an aerobic paddling workout you just make sure to paddle at a pace and intensity that raises your heart rate into your target zone and keeps it there for at least 20 minutes.

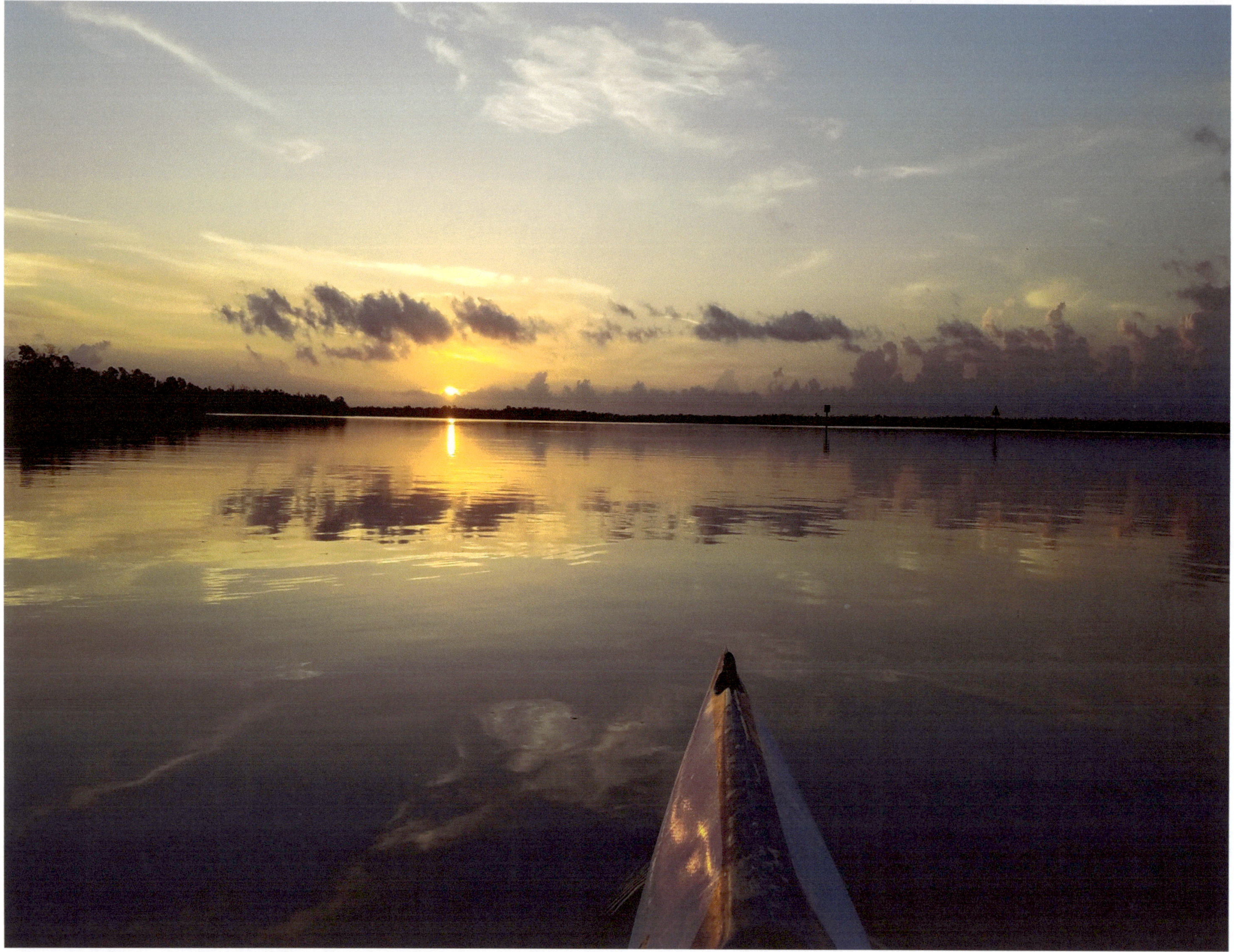

Instructions for Paddling Meditation:

1. Stretch and warm up by paddling gently for a few minutes.

2. If you are interested in getting an aerobic workout, gradually increase your number of strokes/minute until your heart rate is in your aerobic training zone (see running meditation). It is easier to do this if you are wearing a heart rate monitor. If not, you will have to take your pulse while paddling.

3. If you are not interested in getting an aerobic workout just keep up a steady pace for at least 20 minutes (the minimum time needed to achieve a meditative effect).

4. Paddle at this rate for a few minutes and then start to pay attention to your breathing.

5. Count the number of paddle strokes it takes for you to inflate and deflate your lungs.

6. Repeat this number to yourself silently as you continue to paddle at your target pace.

7. Focus on the sensations in your arms, shoulders, torso, hips, legs, and feet as you dip your paddle, pull it back, twist your torso, and drive with your legs.

8. Pay attention to your form as you execute your strokes and maintain your pace.

9. Notice your thoughts and feelings as they enter your consciousness and take you out of the present moment.

10. Tell yourself; "there goes my runaway mind again taking me out of the present moment and into the past or the future."

11. Get refocused on the present moment by synching your breathing with your paddling stroke and counting to yourself.

12. Continue this for at least 20 minutes.

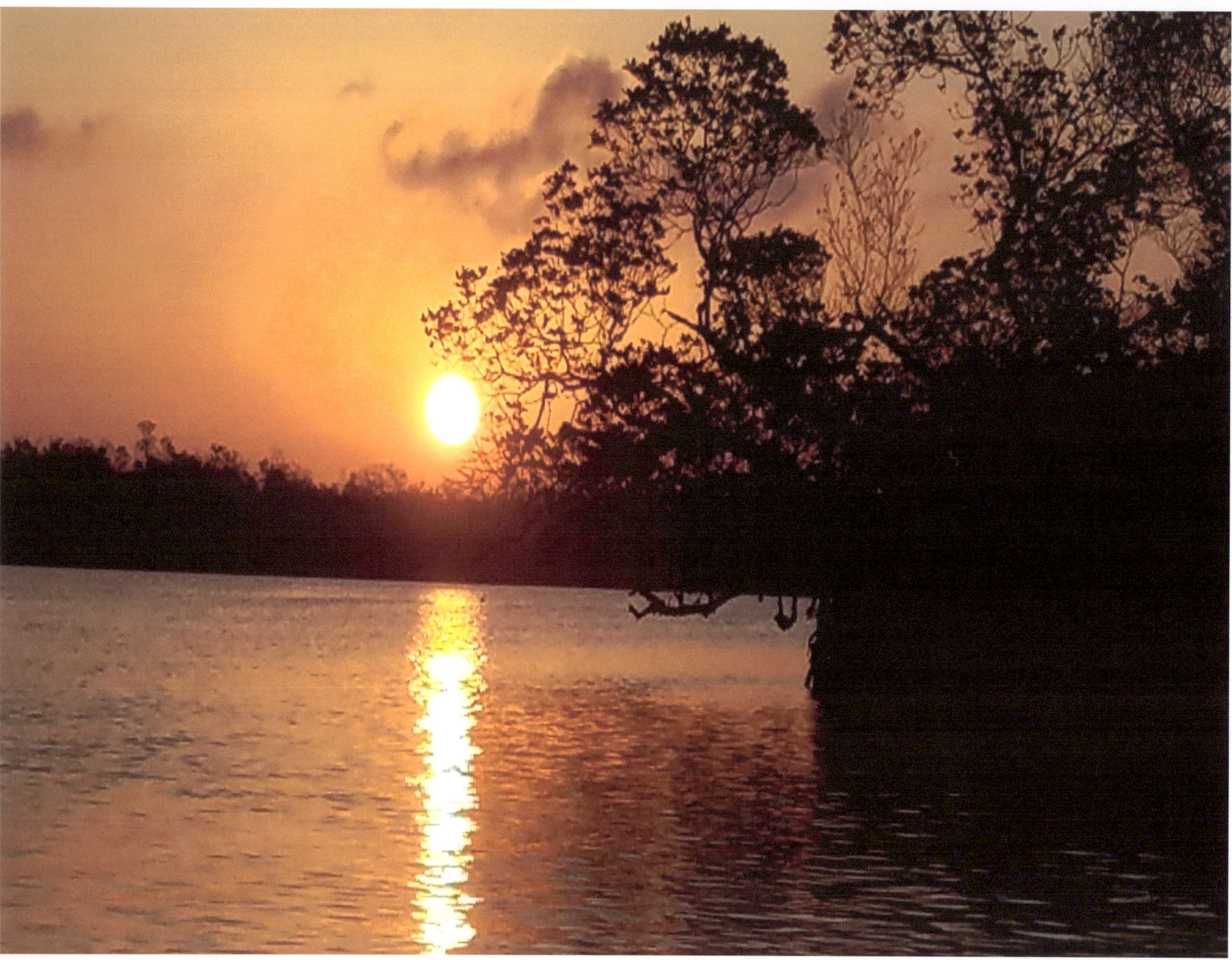

Epilogue

I hope you enjoyed this book and learned a little about mindfulness in the meantime. As I said earlier, it is easy to practice mindfulness on Marco Island. The beauty and majesty of the natural world makes you stop, look, and pay attention. You don't have to live on Marco Island or be a kayaker or runner to reap the rewards of practicing mindfulness. While I've shown how mindfulness can enhance your walking, running, or kayaking, its benefits stretch well beyond the beach or the backwaters. Imagine what your life would be like if you could live it more mindfully with all five senses.

You could:

- Transform your meals into mindful eating experiences bursting with color, flavor, and texture.
- Turn each lovemaking session with your partner into a sensual delight that keeps it new and fresh.
- Turn all your aerobic exercise sessions into moving meditations.
- Listen to music, watch a movie, or read a book with your full attention and focus, appreciating every note, scene, and word.
- Treat each conversation with respect by truly listening to others with understanding.
- Give your work, school. and training activities the full attention and focus they deserve.

These, and other everyday experiences can be made much more rewarding and effective by practicing them more mindfully. Living more mindfully not only enhances your life and helps you get the most out of each experience, it is noticed and appreciated by others. Your boss, spouse/partner, kids, friends and associates will all notice the change in you and respond to you in positive ways you've never experienced before.

Whatever form of mindfulness practice you engage in just remember to enjoy the process. Don't worry about your progress or compare yourself to others. Live mindfully every day and enjoy the beauty of your surroundings wherever you roam.

Dr. Rich Blonna

9 780578 538501